CURVES™

CURVES™

Permanent
Results
Without
Permanent
Dieting

Gary Heavin and Carol Colman

G. P. PUTNAM'S SONS
NEW YORK

Every effort has been made to ensure that the information contained in this book is complete and accurate. However, neither the publisher nor the authors are engaged in rendering professional advice or services to the individual reader. The ideas, procedures, and suggestions contained in this book are not intended as a substitute for consulting with your physician. All matters regarding your health require medical supervision. Neither the authors nor the publisher shall be liable or responsible for any loss or damage allegedly arising from any information or suggestion in this book. The opinions expressed in this book represent the personal views of the authors and not of the publisher.

The recipes contained in this book are to be followed exactly as written. The publisher is not responsible for your specific health or allergy needs that may require medical supervision. The publisher is not responsible for any adverse reactions to the recipes contained in this book.

While the authors have made every effort to provide accurate telephone numbers and Internet addresses at the time of publication, neither the publisher nor the authors assume any responsibility for errors, or for changes that occur after publication.

Penguin Group (USA) Inc. is not associated with Curves, which is solely responsible for the information, services, and products offered herein.

G. P. PUTNAM'S SONS
Publishers Since 1838
a member of
Penguin Group (USA) Inc.
375 Hudson Street
New York, NY 10014

Library of Congress Cataloging-in-Publication Data

Heavin, Gary.
Curves : permanent results without permanent dieting / Gary Heavin and Carol Colman.
p.   cm.
Includes bibliographical references and index.
ISBN 0-399-15061-7 (alk. paper)
1. Women—Health and hygiene.   2. Exercise.   3. Physical fitness.
4. Health.   5. Diet.   6. Nutrition.   I. Colman, Carol.   II. Title.
RA778.H4448   2003   2003043155
613.7'045—dc21

Printed in the United States of America
10   9   8   7   6   5

This book is printed on acid-free paper. ∞

BOOK DESIGN BY DEBORAH KERNER / DANCING BEARS DESIGN
INTERIOR ILLUSTRATIONS BY TANYA MAIBORODA

THIS BOOK IS DEDICATED TO MY
HELPMATE AND WIFE, DIANE. SHE,
LIKE MILLIONS OF OTHER WOMEN
ACROSS THE LAND, DEDICATES HER
LIFE TO THE BENEFIT OF OTHERS.
SHE IS AS BEAUTIFUL ON THE INSIDE
AS SHE IS ON THE OUTSIDE. I
APPRECIATE HER WISDOM AND
INDULGENCE AS SHE SUPPORTS ME
IN MY PURSUIT OF TRUTH.

ACKNOWLEDGMENTS

Much thanks to Susan Petersen Kennedy, Dick Heffernan, Liz Perl, and the entire crew at Putnam for their enthusiasm. A special thanks to Amy Hertz, a terrific editor whose creativity and vision helped make this book a reality, and to Marc Haeringer, a tireless worker who was always there to help us. Gary would like to thank his agent, Janis Vallely, for believing in this project, and Carol would like to thank her agent, Richard Curtis, for his hard work on her behalf.

A special thanks to Cathy Bergin, cofounder of Mean Mommy Publishing, Canon City, Colorado, a cook, food writer, and Curves member who created the wonderful meal plans and recipes used in this book. Cathy and her family follow the Curves meal plan in their own home, and she has made it easy for you to follow it in yours.

We are grateful to researchers Dr. Richard Krieder and Dr. Wayne Westcott, whose searches for truth are inspirational as well as helpful, and to Dr. K. Steven Whiting of the Institute of Nutritional Science, who produced the metabolic testing and many other nutritional considerations for wellness.

We would like to thank exercise physiologist Cassie Findley of Baylor University, who assisted with the home exercise program.

Much thanks to the Curves Sweetheart winners, who shared their stories in this book. These women are truly inspiring.

C O N T E N T S

PART ONE

An End

to Constant

Dieting

CHAPTER 1

THE CURVES PROMISE

Permanent Weight Loss
Without Permanent Dieting

What would you give to have a great body without constantly dieting? Is it worth 30 minutes of your time three days a week? Would you be willing to watch what you eat two days a month if you could eat without deprivation the other 28 days? Would you like to liberate yourself from the drudgery and monotony of constant dieting? I'm going to make you a promise that cannot be made by any other weight-loss program. I will show you an easy way to achieve permanent weight loss without permanent dieting. It won't take a lot of your time. And it will lead you out of diet hell.

I am the CEO and founder of Curves International, which runs fitness centers dedicated to helping women look and feel their best. Our more than 2 million members come from all walks of life, from homemakers to teachers to secretaries to doctors to college athletes. All of them are looking for a fun and effective way to stay fit. They live in big cities like New York, Denver, and Los Angeles, and small towns and suburbs like Sun Valley, Nevada; St. Charles, Missouri; and Naples, Florida. They come to us for a million different reasons. They come because they are tired of living in plus-size bodies, because they are sick of or *sick from* constant dieting. They come because they don't want to show up at their class reunions looking like a swollen version of their former selves, or because they want to be beautiful brides or beautiful mothers of the brides. They come to us because after trying their best on other diets, they have failed. They come to us because on the Curves Weight-Loss and Fitness Program, they succeed. From our inception, we have helped hundreds of thousands of women lose weight, regain their health, and reclaim their lives. I am very proud of the wonderful results our members achieve, and I wish that every woman in the world would join Curves. But that is not why I am writing this book. You don't *have* to be a member of Curves to benefit from the Curves Weight-Loss and Fitness Program. We believe that what we are doing is so important for the health and well-being of women that we want to share it with everyone. And rest assured, you don't even have to belong to any gym or health club to follow the Curves program, because everything I recommend here can be done at home without fancy equipment. This book is designed to help everyone, whether you are an avid exerciser or a beginner who has never done any meaningful physical activity. My program will help you, whether you just need to lose a few pounds or are seriously obese.

What Is Curves?

My wife, Diane, and I opened the first Curves in Harlingen, Texas, in 1992. As of 2003, there are nearly 6,000 Curves in the United States, Canada, Mexico, and Europe, and we will soon be opening Curves in Asia and Australia. We are the fastest-growing franchise in the world—we're even listed in *The Guinness Book of World Records*! Our phenomenal success is not the product of advertising and promotion; rather, it is the result of word-of-mouth recommendations made by happy, slim clients, and you will be reading some of their inspirational stories in this book.

Each Curves offers our unique approach to weight loss, which includes nutritional counseling and an innovative workout that is not only fun but also amazingly effective. We offer two different Curves

Meal Plans that can be customized to suit individual needs. Our members typically lose weight rapidly—and permanently—while following our safe and healthy eating strategies. Our fitness program is incredibly efficient. In just one half-hour, our members can do resistance training, aerobics, and stretching, the three components absolutely essential for fitness, flexibility, and permanent weight loss. I have created a Curves-style workout for women to do at home that is fast, fun, and effective. Those of you who are already Curves members may want to follow the Curves At-Home Workout on days when you can't get to Curves. Curves members who want to continue to get maximum benefit from their Curves workout can follow the tips in Chapter 10, Enhancing Your Workout at Curves.

Taking Care of Yourself Is Not a Luxury

I know that many women reading this book are probably saying to themselves, "Who's got the time for exercise? I barely have time to breathe!" Sadly, seven out of ten Americans don't get regular exercise, and nearly half of all women don't get *any* exercise at all. Exercise is not only good for your figure, it's essential for your health. A sedentary lifestyle increases your risk of developing life-threatening health problems down the road, including heart disease, the number-one killer of women, as well as breast cancer and diabetes. My goal is to make exercise easy and accessible for all women. The truth is, it doesn't take a lot of time to be trim and fit if you exercise efficiently. It just takes commitment and consistency. All I ask is that you devote 30 minutes three times a week to exercise. That's only an hour and a half a week! I understand that many women, between family obligations and work, have no free time. Nevertheless, you must carve out a little amount of time for yourself. Don't think of it as a luxury. You are putting your long-term health at risk if you don't take care of yourself. It's a small investment for a big payoff—a life of good physical and mental health. In combination with the Curves Meal Plan, the right exercise will free you from dieting, once and for all.

Temporary Dieting, Permanent Success

Many of you may be reluctant to embark on a new weight-loss program because you have been disappointed by so many others. If you've failed on other diets, you're not alone. More than 90 percent of all dieters cannot maintain their weight loss for even a year. The reason is simple: Conventional diets set you up for failure. They ask you to do the impossible: diet forever.

Unless you follow these diets for the rest of your life, you'll likely regain your weight. If you don't stay on the diet, within a year or two you typically end up weighing more than you did before you started dieting! So you begin another diet, only this time you find that it's even *harder* to take weight off, so you have to eat even less. And pretty soon, you're sick of the new diet (and sick of being hungry), so you go off it, you gain more weight, and you're back on yet another diet. The vicious cycle begins all over again, each time leaving you a few pounds heavier and weighed down in despair. This phenomenon is so common that it has a name: "the yo-yo syndrome." That's why every major weight-loss plan—from Atkins to the Zone to Weight Watchers—offers a so-called "maintenance diet," a euphemism for *dieting forever.* It's the "small print" in the unspoken contract between dieter and diet. These diets require you to make a lifetime commitment or suffer the consequences. I don't think this is realistic or fair. A diet should be *temporary;* that is, you should be able to go off the diet when you reach your desired weight, and you should be able to do it without regaining those extra pounds that you fought so hard to lose. It should not become a way of life.

There is no maintenance program in this book. I repeat, there is no maintenance program in this book. Once you achieve your goals, you can return to *eating normally most of the time,* not merely on special occasions like your birthday or on designated "days off" from the diet. By *eating normally,* I mean eating 2,500 to 3,000 calories a day, consisting of *real meals* with *real food.* I don't expect you to live on salads or forsake all bread, pizza, soda, and dessert. You don't have to eat like an angel to stay out of diet hell.

When I say you have the freedom to eat normally, it is also my hope that you will chose to eat *healthfully*, at least most of the time. I will give you the latest information on nutrition so that you can stay slim and well. In reality, most of the women who complete my program find themselves eating better because they want to and because when they eat well they feel better and have more energy. But I repeat, you don't have to eat like an angel—you don't have to eat healthfully all the time to succeed.

Unlike standard diets, the Curves Weight-Loss and Fitness Program is designed with the knowledge that you are going to cheat, and there will be times when you may not be able to pass on the french fries, or forgo an ice cream with the kids, and you shouldn't have to pay a steep price for these small pleasures. I will teach you a technique to keep your weight in check. I will give you the tools to maintain your ideal weight for your entire life, without constant deprivation.

Ahead of the Curve

The name "Curves" speaks volumes about our philosophy on health and fitness. Curves conjures the image of femininity, strength, and vitality—not the all-too-common image of rail-thin, unhealthy-looking models living on semi-starvation diets, or that of weak, undernourished women puffing on cigarettes to stay skinny, or that of women who are in the throes of eating disorders because they've been taught to hate their bodies. I am the father of two daughters, and I believe that these images are counterproductive to women's health and their emotional well-being, and that they have done tremendous harm. The success of Curves is proof that you can be strong, lean, and sculpted without starving yourself. Women need not be size 4 or size 6 to look great, as long as they are trim and fit. My mission is to keep you and all women healthy.

I'm not just an entrepreneur. For nearly 30 years, I have been a physical trainer, nutritional counselor, and health club owner. I experienced success early and fast, but it's been a bumpy ride. By the time I was 17, I was pretty much on my own. There were times when I couldn't afford to pay rent and had to sleep in my car, and there were times when I couldn't afford a car and had to sleep on the floor of the health club where I worked. Yet by the time I was 26, I owned seven fitness centers with 25,000 members. I had written a book, *The Sweet Joy of Sugar-Free Living*, which described a dramatic departure from the traditional approach to weight loss. I had made it—I had a loyal following and even my own airplane! Within a few years, I suffered some major financial setbacks and lost everything. Naturally, I was devastated, but in retrospect, that ride up and down was a terrific and necessary learning experience. I continued to work as a fitness trainer, but with more empathy for my clients, many of whom had experienced nothing but disappointment and failure in their lifelong quests to lose weight. The Curves Weight-Loss and Fitness Program is the culmination of nearly three decades of working with thousands of such women.

I'm often asked why I have devoted my life to improving the emotional and physical health of women. From an early age, I understood the importance of women's health and, more important, what happens when women lose their health. When I was 13, my mother, Doris Joy Heavin, who had just turned 40, died of a stroke, leaving behind five children. She was a devoted and loving single mom who was under enormous emotional and financial pressure. For most of her adult life, she suffered from high blood pressure and depression, and was taking lots of medication to no avail. In fact, the drugs just seemed to make her groggy and even more depressed. I now know that conditions such as hers are best treated not by masking symptoms with drugs but by attacking the root cause through dietary changes, exercise, and stress reduction. I've learned that the typical medical model—"diagnose, prescribe drugs, perform surgery"—is the wrong model, and I often think about how the Curves program might have saved her life. But back then, all I knew was that losing her was devastating to me and my siblings. I decided that I wanted to go to medical school so I could help prevent the same tragedy from striking other mothers and their children. I worked my way through two years of college, following a pre-med curriculum that included courses in biology and human physiology. The courses gave me a wonderful grounding in science, but before I could graduate, I was forced to drop out of school to work full-time. I took over a failing health club, which gave me a welcome opportunity to make money while helping people avoid getting sick in the first place. Still, I never gave up my goal of finishing school. Later in life, despite my busy work schedule, I earned my BS in Health and Nutritional Counseling from Thomas Edison State College in New Jersey.

My deep faith helped me get through some difficult times. I'm a born-again Christian, and I take my commitment to God and humanity very seriously. My wife, Diane, and I believe that we have been blessed, and we believe that to whom much is given, much is expected. Among our many projects, we are currently funding research at Baylor University in Texas that will test my weight-loss theories in a research environment.

The Conventional Wisdom Didn't Work

I loved working as a trainer and was deeply committed to making a positive difference in the lives of my clients. Early in my career, however, I was disturbed by the fact that the standard dietary advice of "eat less to lose weight" didn't make sense for most women. I observed that although many women were already on strict, low-calorie diets, they were not only not losing weight—over time, they were gaining weight. Inevitably, out of frustration, they would go off their diets, gain even more weight, and then go on another diet. They were the victims of a vicious diet cycle. Each time they lost and gained weight, the pounds became increasingly harder to lose. I concluded that the standard weight-loss programs being followed by my clients were hopelessly flawed. The reason seemed obvious. Typical low-calorie diets wreak havoc on metabolism, the process by which the nutrients in food are broken down into smaller particles that can be made into energy to run the body. Simply put, the body uses up the nutrients it needs to do work and stores excess nutrients primarily as fat. But that's not the end of the story. I knew that there was much more involved in metabolism than simply "calories in, calories burned." I observed that pregnant women seem to gain weight even when they suffer bouts of morning sickness and eat little food. It became obvious to me that hormones could influence metabolism—for better or for worse—a fact that was ignored by conventional diets.

I reached the conclusion that dieting turns on so-called "starvation hormones" that actually enable the body to survive on less food and burn less energy. There is a good biological reason for this. If the human body could not adapt and live on fewer calories, our ancestors would have perished during times of famine. Thus, our bodies are naturally trained to go into "starvation mode" when we reduce our intake of calories. When this happens, we *lower* our metabolic rate, which means that we do more with less. For our ancestors, this meant survival. For 21st-century dieters, this mechanism means a vicious and endless cycle. Over time, because they are very efficient, our bodies learn how to function on fewer and fewer calories, and we continually keep lowering our metabolic rate. This means that we have to eat less to maintain the same weight and eat *much* less to lose weight. It also means that if we resume eating a normal number of calories, we will gain more weight back.

Dieting not only triggers the production of starvation hormones, but low-fat, low-calorie dieting also sabotages a woman's metabolism in another way. When you diet, the goal is to lose fat, not muscle. Why? Fat is what makes you look lumpy and flabby. Muscle is what makes you look trim and lean. In fact, many women find that when they lose fat and gain muscle, they look slimmer, even if they haven't lost a pound! But the loss of muscle does more than affect how you look. It also has a devastating impact on your metabolism.

Muscle is the most metabolically active tissue in the body. A pound of muscle burns as much as 50 calories a day *at rest*. That means that when you are sleeping, or sitting at your desk, or driving your car, your muscles are burning calories. Thus, muscle is a good thing, and something you want as much of as possible, but muscle is hard to keep. As we age, we lose five to ten pounds of muscle each decade, primarily due to inactivity. We accelerate muscle loss by dieting. You may be shocked to learn that on most low-fat, low-calorie diets, you lose substantial amounts of muscle along with the fat. In fact, if you manage to lose 20 pounds on a diet, you may have lost up to eight pounds of muscle. As you lose muscle, your metabolic rate decreases further, the result being that you have to eat a lot less to stay slim. Every time you diet, you lose more muscle and lower your metabolism yet again. Clearly, typical low-fat, low-calorie dieting can have disastrous consequences. If you stay on a low-fat, low-calorie, low-protein diet for an extended period of time, you will lose muscle, destroy your metabolism, and compromise your health.

The Missing Link in Weight Loss

There is an alternative to the standard low-calorie diet, and I have been teaching it to my clients for years. It is the same program that has made Curves the success it is today. There is one big difference between the Curves Weight-Loss and Fitness Program and other weight-loss programs. Unlike other weight-loss plans, my program is designed to raise the metabolic rate, so that as you follow the program, *your metabolism actually increases,* allowing you to eat more food without gaining weight. In other words, you lose unwanted pounds, but not by paying the price of perpetually lower metabolism. My program achieves this increase in metabolism without causing unwanted weight gain and without triggering the starvation response that makes conventional dieting a frustrating exercise in futility. That's why you're able to resume normal eating after reaching your desired weight, and that's why you don't have to spend the rest of your life on a diet.

The truth, however, is that dieting alone will not restore your metabolism. Why? Remember that when you follow a conventional diet, you often lose a substantial amount of muscle, and muscle is what burns calories. In order to achieve permanent weight loss, you have to increase your muscle mass so that you keep burning calories efficiently. There is only one way to do this, and that is strength training. You need to lift weights or use other exercise equipment that forces you to work your muscles against resistance. You've heard the expression "Use it or lose it"? It's especially true for muscle. In order to protect or make more muscle, you need to use your muscles. You need to work them hard until they fatigue. Bigger muscles create a smaller body. You know the actresses that you see on television who have slim, sculpted, defined bodies? They're all doing some form of strength training. If you don't do it, you can't achieve permanent weight loss, and any diet guru who tells you otherwise is lying. Sure, you'll lose weight on any low-calorie diet, but you will be stuck in diet hell unless you protect your metabolism, and the only way to do that is to add muscle. You don't have to spend hours working out to increase muscle mass; 30 minutes three times a week is all it takes.

Nearly 30 years ago, I was one of the first trainers to advocate weight training for women. When I first began insisting that my clients work with weights or on machines, I had to spend hours convincing them that they weren't going to become muscle-bound, unattractive women. Trust me: No matter how hard a woman works out, her body doesn't make enough male hormones for her to ever look like a guy. Once my skeptical clients started seeing amazing results, they stopped resisting. Not only did they lose fat and develop muscle tone practically overnight, but the real payoff came when they could stop dieting, eat normally and healthfully, and not gain the weight back.

Women often ask me whether they still have to do strength training if they go to aerobics class or walk. The answer is an emphatic yes. Although aerobics and walking are great for your heart, they do not build muscle. In fact, if you're doing a lot of aerobics and you're on a typical low-calorie diet, you may chew up even more muscle than you would lose just by dieting alone! Aerobic exercise without weight training could actually undermine your efforts to achieve permanent weight loss.

The Curves Weight-Loss and Fitness Program

The Curves Weight-Loss and Fitness Program has three components, each of which works in synergy with the others to help slim and tone your body while resetting your metabolism.

- The Curves Meal Plan
- The Curves Workout
- The Curves Supplement Regimen

The Curves Meal Plan

The Curves Meal Plan reprograms your metabolism to work for you, not against you. It is designed to correct the disastrous effects of years of low-fat, low-calorie starvation diets and yo-yo dieting. You will choose between two different meal plans, each designed to accommodate different metabolic needs. The first meal plan, the Carbohydrate-Sensitive Plan, is a high-protein, low-carbohydrate meal plan for those of you who are carbohydrate-intolerant. The second, the Calorie-Sensitive Plan, is designed for those of you who are not good candidates for the advantages of a high-protein meal plan. I will explain the difference between these two plans in Chapters 2 and 3. In Chapter 3, I have also provided a short quiz that will help you determine which meal plan you should follow. Both meal plans are divided into three phases.

- **PHASE 1 · GET OFF TO A GREAT START.** The first phase is the strictest phase of the program. It jump-starts your weight loss by shifting your body into fat-burning mode. Most women lose 6 to 10 pounds fairly quickly. Phase 1 is the most restrictive part of the diet, but you are only on it for one or two weeks, depending on how much weight you need to lose.

- **PHASE 2 · REACH YOUR GOAL.** In Phase 2, you are eating considerably more food but still losing weight (about one to two pounds per week). You stay on Phase 2 until you reach your desired weight, hit a plateau, or need a break from dieting.

- **PHASE 3 · RETRAIN YOUR METABOLISM.** Phase 3 is the fulfillment of the Curves Promise: permanent weight loss without permanent dieting. In Phase 3, you are no longer on a diet. On most days, you will be eating between 2,500 and 3,000 calories, yet you will keep the weight off. You will learn how and why this is possible in Chapter 2, Metabolic Magic: Escaping the Diet Trap of Slow Metabolism.

I understand how busy women are today, so my goal is to make this program as easy to follow as possible. In Chapters 5 and 6, you will find seven weeks of Curves Meal Plan sample menus, so you'll never run out of ideas about what to eat. In the Curves Daily Planner, starting on page 253, I also provide weekly shopping lists, recipes, and charts to help you plan your meals and track your progress. I promise, following this Curves Meal Plan is not going to be a chore. And don't worry, you won't even have to prepare different meals for your family. As you will see, it's easy to stay on your meal plan and still satisfy your family without a lot of extra work.

The Curves Workout

The Curves At-Home Workout will help build new calorie-burning muscle while you slim down and tone up. The 30-minute regimen is a combination of strength training, aerobics, and stretching. I show you how to do a complete upper- and lower-body workout while exercising your cardiovascular system at the same time. The workout is efficient, effective, and enjoyable. The only equipment you need is a simple, inexpensive exercise resistance tube you can buy at any discount department store or sporting-goods store, or even on the Internet. The best news is that you only need to do these exercises three times a week to achieve spectacular results. My program is designed to accommodate the needs of women regardless of their level of fitness. It enables you to go at your own pace. Don't miss the free week at Curves coupon at the back of this book.

The Curves Supplement Regimen

Most of us do not get all the nutrients we need from food alone. Modern food-processing techniques have stripped the vitamins, minerals, and other beneficial chemicals out of the food supply, while adding tons of preservatives, insecticides, food dyes, and other chemicals that are foreign to our bodies. Nutrient deficiency can sabotage your weight-loss efforts by promoting food cravings and making you feel tired. In

Chapter 11, I provide information on nutritional supplements that can help ensure that you are getting the nutrients your body needs. This is important, because even careful eaters may be nutrient deficient, and those you of who are not so careful are particularly at risk.

Reclaiming Your Health

Chapter 12, Special Health Concerns: The Curves Solutions, explains how the basic Curves principles of good nutrition, exercise, nutritional supplements, and revitalization of the spirit can help prevent and treat several health issues that affect women. These issues include arthritis, diabetes, heart disease, menopause, osteoporosis, and pregnancy. I provide a guide for women who have special health concerns that may make them reluctant to embark on a fitness regimen. I address the particular needs of these women and show how, with the cooperation of their physicians, they can incorporate fitness and nutrition into their lives.

Within the pages of this book, you will find the tools you need to liberate yourself from the tyranny of perpetual dieting, unhealthy lifestyles, and many chronic illnesses. Whether you have struggled with a weight problem all of your life or are just trying to shed a few pounds that you only recently acquired, the Curves program will enable you to achieve your goals safely, quickly, effectively, and *permanently.*

Curves Profile

CONNIE W.

FARMINGTON, MISSOURI

From my 20s on, I had been fighting with my weight. I also had a weight problem when I was a child, but I managed to take off the extra pounds when I got into sports in junior high and high school.

In my 20s, I stopped exercising and started gaining. Before I knew it, I was in my early 40s and I wore a size 20. I was 5'5" tall and weighed 208 pounds. I was under a great deal of stress working full-time and pursuing a doctorate in educational leadership. I enjoyed the challenge of my hectic schedule, but I had completely neglected my health. I had terrible eating habits, and I hadn't done any exercise since I was a teenager. I would get tired just walking up a flight of steps. I coached the cheerleading squad, but I couldn't go out on the field and do anything with them. I could only tell them what to do. In February 2000, I had a wake-up call—literally. I received a phone call from a high school classmate inviting me to my 25th reunion. I didn't want to go looking the way I did.

That call gave me the incentive to make some positive life changes. I decided to join Curves. At first, I was worried that I would not be able to keep up with the exercises, but once I began, I realized that the program was designed to meet the needs of everyone: people like me, who had not exercised in years, as well as women who were fit. The best part, as far as I was concerned, was that it was a 30-minute workout that I could easily incorporate into my daily schedule. I followed the Curves Meal Plan, and by the time I went to my reunion at the end of June, I had lost 40 pounds. But I still had more to lose.

A real challenge came in the summer of 2000, when I had to live on campus for the month of July to complete my doctorate. That meant I was four hours away from home and basically living out of a suitcase. Fortunately, there was a Curves in the university town and I was able to continue my fitness program.

It took me about a year to lose all the weight I needed to lose. I am now 75 pounds lighter and wear a size 2 or 4. I have maintained my current weight for almost two years. My energy level has soared, my self-confidence and my self-respect have returned, and I am happier and more easygoing in every aspect of my life. To me, Curves isn't just about looking good. Everyone sees the external change, but my husband and I see the internal change. I'm happier than I have been in years, and people tell me that they think I'm more outgoing. Obviously, I go out a lot more and do more things than I used to do because I'm more comfortable with myself. In addition, I don't get as tired.

I am a Health and Family and Consumer Science teacher and a student council adviser. When I was heavier, I would stand up in front of the classroom and think to myself, *I'm such a horrible role model. How can I stand up here and tell these kids what they should be doing when I'm not doing it myself?* I can speak truthfully from the heart now instead of saying "Do as I say, not as I do." Curves has helped me become a positive role model for my students, and I'm proud that I am setting a good example for them.

CHAPTER 2

METABOLIC MAGIC

Escaping the Diet Trap
of Slow Metabolism

As every dieter knows, losing weight is the easy part. Keeping it off is the real challenge. Most people never succeed—as soon as they go off the diet, they regain the weight they lost and then some. The fault is not with the dieter, it's with the diet. Conventional diets ignore the fact that dieting is an unnatural state and that the human body responds in ways that can sabotage your best efforts. You want to lose fat; your body desperately tries to hold on to it. You want to burn more calories than you are consuming; your body tricks you by running on fewer calories. At the end of your struggle, what do you have to show for all your hard work? A slower metabolism, which forces you to eat less and less to stay slim.

How is the Curves Weight-Loss and Fitness Program different from standard diets? By the time you have completed the program, you will have achieved a feat impossible on other diets. You will have raised, not lowered, your metabolism. You will be able to eat a normal amount—between 2,500 and 3,000 calories a day—without putting on unwanted pounds. You will go from a food-burning machine to a champion fat-burning machine, and you will escape the diet trap of slow metabolism.

The Curves Weight-Loss and Fitness Program will retrain your metabolism to work for you, not against you. You will finally be able to shed the excess weight and keep it off without starving yourself. You will be able to fulfill the Curves Promise—permanent weight loss without permanent dieting.

How is it possible to lose weight and not have to starve yourself for the rest of your life to stay slim? The secret to our success is that we address the complicated biological issues that have been conveniently overlooked by conventional diets. Simply telling people to eat less, as most diets do, will not overcome the hurdles that prevent permanent weight loss. The only way to achieve real and long-lasting results is to anticipate these problems and to have a good offense ready to deal with them.

We also recognize that the "one size fits all" approach to weight loss simply does not work. That's why we offer two different meal plans. The first, the Carbohydrate-Sensitive Plan, is for people who are carbohydrate-intolerant—that is, they have eaten too many carbohydrates for too long. Carbohydrate-sensitive people can eat all the protein foods they need and still lose weight. The second meal plan, the Calorie-Sensitive Plan, is for people who can only lose weight the old-fashioned way—by counting calories. These people can actually *gain* weight on high-protein diets and should avoid them. (Take the tests on pages 41–42 to see which plan is the right one for you.)

Although most women will succeed on either the Carbohydrate-Sensitive Plan or the Calorie-Sensitive Plan, not everyone responds the same way. Some women may need to switch from one plan to another to get better results. Others may find that they are too tired on a very low-carbohydrate or low-calorie regimen, and they may need to adjust their food intake accordingly. Therefore, we provide specific information on how you can tailor either meal plan to better suit your individual needs.

Do You Need a Metabolic Tune-Up?

Unlike other diets, we acknowledge that there are some overweight people who should *not* try to lose weight, at least not yet. These people have destroyed their metabolism through years of low-fat, low-calorie or yo-yo dieting and bombarding their bodies with the wrong food. No matter how much they cut calories or restrict carbohydrates, their metabolism is too low. Metabolic Magic cannot happen until these women repair their "broken" metabolism and restore it to normal function. Some of you may already know that you fall into this category, others will find out shortly after you begin dieting. The good news is that there is a simple solution to your problem. It's called the Metabolic Tune-Up (see page 35). It's an easy way to prime your metabolism so that you can finally achieve permanent weight loss. You stay on the Metabolic Tune-Up for two to three months, or as long as it takes to reinvigorate your metabolism.

PROBLEM 1: **Your Hormones Are Working Against You**

The human body was designed to live in a completely different environment than the one in which we live today. Our prehistoric ancestors were hunter-gatherers who alternated between times of feast and times of famine. During the warm months, when food was abundant, our ancestors would gorge on fresh meat, seeds, roots, nuts, fruits, and berries. (Take note: When they wanted to put on body fat, they ate carbs along with protein and fat.) In the winter, when food was scarce, they lived primarily on dried meat and whatever else they could forage. And sometimes they went without food for days at a time and survived due to stored body fat. Fortunately, when food was in short supply, their bodies adapted by requiring less energy.

Modern men and women may be light years ahead of our prehistoric ancestors intellectually, but the fact is, we still have the same bodies and the same metabolism. And when you go on a diet and cut back on your intake of calories, you trigger the same biochemical response. In fact, about 72 hours after starting a typical weight-loss program, your body begins to produce hormones—so-called "starvation hormones"—that resist burning fat. Over time, your body becomes more efficient and requires fewer calories to do the same amount of work. Inevitably, your metabolism slows down so that you, like your prehistoric ancestors, can run on less energy. This may have been great for them, but it has created untold misery for millions of modern dieters. When you're off the weight-loss program, you are stuck with a slower metabolism than when you started, so you will begin to rapidly gain weight when you start eating more food.

CURVES SOLUTION: **Control Starvation Hormones**

Most diets keep you on the same low-fat, low-calorie regimen until you reach your desired weight.

On the Curves Meal Plan, you are never on a very low-calorie regimen for more than two weeks at a time. This helps limit the accumulation of starvation hormones that would otherwise bring your metabolism down to a slow crawl. After Phase 1—the most restrictive part of the program but also the shortest—you will eat an ample amount of food but still lose weight. This ramps up your metabolism so that you are not locked in a losing battle with your body. (If your starvation hormones do kick in while you are dieting, as they are programmed to do, you need a Metabolic Tune-Up, as I will discuss later.)

PROBLEM 2:   **The Dreaded Mid-Diet Plateau**

There's nothing more disappointing than when you lose weight for the first few weeks or months that you're on a diet, and then, even though you are doing everything right, you suddenly stop losing weight before you have reached your goal. This phenomenon is so common that there's a name for it: "the plateau." How do conventional diets deal with the plateau? They tell you to stay on the same diet but eat less or increase your exercise! That's precisely the wrong advice, because it ignores the reason you've reached a plateau in the first place. While you've been losing weight, you've been living on stored energy. As you deplete your fat stores, your body responds by trying to protect you from starvation. Your starvation hormones kick in and lower your metabolism so that you can live on less energy. Once again, you must control your starvation hormones before you can start to lose weight.

CURVES SOLUTION: **Eat More to Lose More**

When you reach a plateau, *you eat more, not less.* That's right. Forget the conventional wisdom. That's what got you into this mess in the first place. The only way to jump-start your metabolism is to stoke it with more food. You need a Metabolic Tune-Up, not a low-calorie tune-down. Depending on your metabolism, over time the starvation hormones will dissipate, your metabolism will become unstuck, and you will be able to resume your weight-loss plan until you reach your goal.

PROBLEM 3: **Dieting Chews Up Your Muscle**

You've undoubtedly heard that for every 3,500 calories you carve out of your diet, you will lose a pound of fat. The problem is, it's not true. You will lose one pound, but it isn't all fat. In fact, if you are following the conventional low-calorie, high-carbohydrate diet, up to a third of all the weight you are losing is *muscle.* Losing muscle will make it extremely difficult for you to maintain your desired weight. Muscle is much more metabolically active than fat—muscle burns more calories, even when you are not exercising. Thus, the loss of muscle further lowers your metabolism, condemning you to diet hell forever. Muscle is also important because it supports your bones and joints, and keeps you standing straight and strong. If you lose muscle, you are more likely to develop orthopedic problems such as osteoarthritis and osteoporosis, which can limit your physical activity and will make it even harder to maintain your weight loss.

CURVES SOLUTION: **Make More Muscle**

The Curves Weight-Loss and Fitness Program is specifically designed not only to prevent muscle loss but to *increase* muscle mass. Both the Carbohydrate-Sensitive and Calorie-Sensitive versions of the Curves Meal Plan have adequate protein to both protect existing muscle and build new muscle. Protein provides the body with amino acids, which are essential for cell growth and repair. Amino acids are stored in your muscle cells. If your body is not getting enough protein in your diet, it will drain the amino acids from your muscle to use in other parts of your body. The end result is that you may be losing weight, but you are also losing muscle, which will make you look flabbier. So eat your protein!

The Curves Workout, specifically the weight-training component, further strengthens and builds muscle. When you follow the Curves Meal Plan and do the workout, you will lose all your unwanted weight in the form of fat, gain more calorie-burning muscle, and develop a well-toned, sculpted body.

PROBLEM 4: You're Fighting Hunger and Food Cravings

It's unreasonable to expect anyone to stick to a meal plan if they are constantly feeling hungry and deprived. Ultimately, you will fail if a meal plan is too hard to follow. Most popular weight-loss diets are too restrictive in either the amount or variety of food that they allow. Many high-protein diets require that you go for weeks or months without ever eating a piece of real bread or a piece of fruit. Most high-carbohydrate, low-fat, low-calorie diets are too low in protein, which means that dieters on those plans will be constantly hungry.

CURVES SOLUTION: More Food, More Variety, More Often

Both versions of the Curves Meal Plan contain ample amounts of protein and fat so you won't feel hungry, while allowing you to eat generous amounts of healthy carbohydrates so you won't get bored. At the same time, we limit (but do not ban) starchy carbohydrates and fruit. If you want a piece of bread, or a serving of pasta, or a piece of fruit, you can have it as long as you do not exceed the day's carbohydrate allowance for Phases 1 or 2. In my experience, women are more likely to succeed on the Curves Meal Plan because it offers enough food and enough variety.

On the Curves Meal Plan, you eat six small meals a day rather than the traditional three large meals. This provides a steady stream of fuel so you don't get ravenous and are less likely to succumb to cravings. If you do feel like munching on something, you can eat an unlimited amount of the Free Foods (see Free Foods list, page 57), the high-fiber vegetables that fill you up quickly and provide incredible health benefits. You can also have one delicious protein shake daily, which is a great replacement for dessert (see page 59).

PROBLEM 5: The Post-Diet Rebound

On most other diets, once you have reached your desired weight, you graduate to a so-called "maintenance" program that you must follow for the rest of your life to keep the weight off. When you start eating normally, as you inevitably will, you will gain the weight back. The diet gurus blame you for "reverting to your old habits." What they don't tell you is that they're to blame for your problems. Their diets have lowered your metabolism so that it runs on fewer calories. You are trapped in diet hell!

The goal of the Curves Weight-Loss and Fitness Program is to achieve your desired weight so that you can *stop dieting*. In Chapter 1, I promised that if you are willing to watch what you eat one or two days a month, you will be able to eat normally the other 28. Now I will explain how we perform this feat of magic.

CURVES SOLUTION: The Phase 3 Miracle

Phase 3 is not a diet or a maintenance program. It is a tool to ramp up your metabolism so that you will be able to eat normally for the rest of your life. Compared to conventional diets, the Curves Weight-Loss and Fitness Program will leave your metabolism in better shape, because you burned mostly fat and not muscle. In fact, most of you will gain muscle on my program. Nevertheless, while you are on any weight-loss program, you will eat less food than normal, which will have a dampening effect on your metabolic rate, and you will still have to rid your body of some starvation hormones. You need to retrain your metabolism to burn more energy. The happy solution is that you get to eat more food!

When you start Phase 3, you will increase your food intake to about

2,500 to 3,000 calories a day. You don't have to eat any special way—
you no longer have to count carbohydrate grams and calories. If, however, counting calories helps you initially figure out what 2,500 to 3,000
calories should be, by all means do so. You will weigh yourself every day
and keep track of your weight on the Phase 3 Chart in your Curves
Daily Planner. Initially, you will find that you are regaining weight
fairly rapidly, which is normal. Some of that new weight is water—
about two to three pounds—because your body throws off water when
you begin a diet and puts water back on when you go off a diet. Anything above that, however, is fat. As soon as you regain about three to
five pounds, you go back on Phase 1 to burn off the fat. Within a day or
two, you should be back to your low weight—that is, the weight you
were when you began Phase 3. Then you resume eating normally and
healthfully, and you will regain some weight, but this time it takes a bit
longer. When you regain three to five pounds, you go back on Phase 1
to burn it off. Each time you repeat this cycle, you will see that it takes
longer and longer to put on the weight. The key is to *not* gain more
weight than you can lose in 72 hours, before those starvation hormones
kick in again. Eventually, when your metabolism is raised, you can eat
normally for a month or so at a time before you have to go back on
Phase 1 to burn off any unwanted fat.

Do you have to eat a healthy diet? I believe many of you will make
better food choices than when you started, but it is not a requirement.

There are two things that you need to understand for Phase 3 to make
sense: (1) how eating affects your metabolism, and (2) how people gain
weight. When you understand these two points, you will understand how
you can eat normally and not gain weight.

More Food = Faster Metabolism

Three decades ago, when I saw my clients reaching plateaus on their
diets, I intuitively realized that they needed to eat more food to stimulate their metabolism. Paradoxically, when I told them to increase their
caloric intake for a few weeks, they were finally able to go back on the
diet and start losing weight again. This is not just a personal observa-

tion, it is a scientific fact. My experience with thousands of clients was validated in 1995 by a groundbreaking scientific study published in the *New England Journal of Medicine,* which showed that metabolism shifts up and down depending on daily food intake. As I had noted decades earlier, metabolism decreases when people eat less but *increases when people eat more.* In fact, if you feed people 2,500 calories daily, their metabolic rates will eventually adapt to the increase in food. We all know people who can seemingly eat as much as they want yet not gain weight. They have acquired their higher metabolism by eating lots of food. One day, you may be able to do the same thing. In Phase 3, when I ask you to eat 2,500 to 3,000 calories daily, don't be afraid to do it. Your metabolism will eventually rise to the challenge.

Weight Gain: Slow but Steady

You've undoubtedly heard the expression, "If we don't understand the mistakes of the past, we are condemned to repeat them." When it comes to weight loss, it is right on target. If you want to keep excess weight off, you need to understand how you put it on in the first place. Women often complain that they feel like they ballooned from a size 8 to a size 16 practically overnight, but this is usually not the case. In reality, for most women, it has been a slow and steady rise up the scale, as the weight creeps on insidiously, month after month, year after year. Only after you reach a critical mass—that is, you're about 30 pounds overweight—do you notice how the weight crept on through the years. Studies show that people typically gain six pounds a year, which culminates in a 30-pound gain over five years. Thirty pounds sounds like a lot of weight, but in reality, it breaks down to an increase of only half a pound or so every month. I ask you: How long does it take you to lose half a pound? If you had done nothing different over the past five years except diet one or two days a month, would you still be overweight today? The answer is NO!

Most people are willing to diet for the one or two days a month it takes to lose a few pounds, in exchange for the freedom of eating normally the rest of the time. This is the fundamental strategy behind Phase 3. In Phase 3, you do not allow yourself to gain more than three to five pounds at a time. When you gain this weight, you go back to Phase 1 to quickly remove it. At first, many of you will find yourself back in Phase 1 within a few days, but eventually you will have increased your metabolism so that you can eat normally most of the time and still maintain your desired weight. Once you have mastered Phase 3, you will be free from perpetual dieting, and you will have the tools and the skill to stay slim forever.

Making the Metabolic Miracle Work for You: Three Phases to Permanent Weight Loss

Now that you understand the underlying principles of the Curves Weight-Loss and Fitness Program, I want to show you how to make the metabolic miracle work for you. The Curves Meal Plan consists of three phases, each phase building on the success of the others to achieve your goal of *no more permanent dieting!*

Phase 1

GOALS: **RAPID WEIGHT LOSS**
LEARN HOW TO CONTROL YOUR WEIGHT
GET OFF TO A GREAT START!

HOW LONG: **NO MORE THAN TWO WEEKS**

Whether you are on the Carbohydrate-Sensitive Plan or the Calorie-Sensitive Plan, Phase 1 is the strictest part of the program. It is also the shortest.

- If you want to lose less than 20 pounds, follow Phase 1 for only one week.
- If you want to lose more than 20 pounds, stay on Phase 1 for two weeks.
- When you are finished with Phase 1, move on to Phase 2.

Women on the Carbohydrate-Sensitive Plan can eat unlimited amounts of protein (including lean meats, cheeses, eggs, seafood, and poultry), but *no more than 20 grams of carbohydrates.* In addition, you are allowed unlimited amounts of Free Foods and one protein shake daily. (See Free Foods on page 57.) If you are on the Carbohydrate-Sensitive Plan, you must drink at least eight glasses of water daily, which, by the way, is a good idea for everyone. In Chapter 5, you will find sample menus for Phase 1 and Phase 2 on the Carbohydrate-Sensitive Plan. Use your Daily Meal Planner on pages 311–16 to help you keep track of your daily carbohydrate consumption.

Women on the Calorie-Sensitive Plan eat *1,200 calories* daily and no more than *60 grams of carbohydrates* in Phase 1. Try to consume about 40 percent of your daily calories from protein. Be sure to stick to the correct protein portion sizes or you'll risk eating too many calories. You are also allowed to eat unlimited amounts of Free Foods and one protein shake daily. (See Free Foods on page 57.) In Chapter 6, you will find sample menus for Phase 1 and Phase 2 on the Calorie-Sensitive Plan. Use your Daily Meal Planner on pages 311–16 to help you keep track of both your calorie and carbohydrate intake.

KEEPING TRACK · How do you know how many calories or carbohydrates are in a particular food? Read the label. Packaged foods will list the calorie and carbohydrate content of the average serving size. But not all foods come in packages. In Chapter 4, you will find a list of the carbohydrate and calorie content of commonly consumed foods. I also recommend that you buy a food guide, such as Corinne T. Netzer's *Complete Book of Food Counts,* which includes the carbohydrate and calorie counts (and other vital information) for a wide variety of fresh and packaged foods. When you are calculating the carbs and calories in your meal, don't forget to subtract the amount of carbs and calories in any Free Foods that you've included, because they don't count toward your totals.

Phase 1 provides instant gratification: Most women lose about 4 to 6 pounds—some lose as much as 10 pounds in two weeks—and are thrilled with the results. It is also a wonderful confidence builder. It gives you the tools and the ability to lose weight rapidly when you need to, which will come in handy during Phase 3.

Some of you may be so happy with your results on Phase 1 that you may be tempted to stay in this phase for longer than you should. Please don't. It is imperative that you move on to Phase 2 at the right time, for several reasons. First, you don't want your metabolism to get used to running on such a low-calorie or low-carbohydrate diet. The fact is, as motivated as you may be, it is extremely difficult to stick to such a strict eating plan for any length of time. Second, Phase 1 does not include a wide enough variety of nutrients that are essential for a healthy body. It's impossible to get an adequate amount of essential vitamins, minerals, and other beneficial nutrients on a mere 1,200 calories a day. A week or two on a low-calorie regimen is fine, but staying on that regimen any longer than that is not in your best interest. Remember, Curves is not just about being slim for life—it's about staying healthy for life. You shouldn't have to sacrifice your health to be thin, and you don't need to. To make sure that you are getting enough nutrients, I urge you to take a multivitamin/mineral supplement daily. (See Chapter 11, Total Health Supplements for Enhancing the Curves Program.)

PROBLEM: What If You Don't Lose Enough?
Although most women will lose a substantial amount of weight during Phase 1, a small minority may not. Don't get frustrated. There is a simple solution to this problem.

- If you are on the Calorie-Sensitive Plan and you have not lost at least three pounds during the first week and two pounds in the second week, your metabolism is stuck in low gear. You need to turn it up before you can lose weight. The solution? The Metabolic Tune-Up, during which you will eat more food to get your metabolism moving again. (See page 35.)
- If you are on the Carbohydrate-Sensitive Plan and have not lost at least three pounds during the first week and two pounds the second week, switch to the Calorie-Sensitive Plan. If

within a week you still haven't lost at least three pounds, go to the Metabolic Tune-Up for a metabolic adjustment. (See page 35.)

PROBLEM: Too Tired to Function

Some women may find that they are very tired during Phase 1 and are literally dragging themselves through the day. There's a reason for this. Whether you are on the Carbohydrate-Sensitive Plan or the Calorie-Sensitive Plan, your metabolism must adjust to your new way of eating. You are now forcing your metabolism to change from a food-burning machine to a fat-burning machine, for which the primary fuel is stored energy. This transition may be more difficult for some of you than for others. For example, true carbohydrate addicts on the Carbohydrate-Sensitive Plan may find that their blood sugar dips too low at 20 grams of carbohydrates, causing headaches, dizziness, and other unpleasant symptoms. I don't want you to feel miserable! If you can't get through the day, please increase your carbohydrate intake to *40 grams daily*. You will feel much better, and it should not interfere with your weight loss. Your metabolism is so used to functioning on very high amounts of carbohydrates that the extra 20 grams is a drop in the bucket. Your metabolism will hardly notice that it's there. Within a few days, once you've adjusted to fewer carbohydrates, you can try reducing your carbohydrate intake to 20 grams. If you feel fine on the lower amount, you can continue on 20 grams throughout Phase 1. If not, go back up to 40 grams until you are ready to start Phase 2.

If you are feeling excessively tired on the Calorie-Sensitive Plan at 1,200 calories, move on to Phase 2, where you will increase your caloric intake to 1,600. Most women find that this does the trick: They feel reenergized but can still lose weight.

Phase 2

GOAL: **LOSE ONE OR TWO POUNDS OF FAT EACH WEEK**

HOW LONG: **UNTIL YOU REACH YOUR DESIRED WEIGHT, OR YOU PLATEAU, OR YOU NEED A BREAK FROM THE PROGRAM**

During Phase 2, you eat more food and a greater variety of food. It is more satisfying than Phase 1 and not very difficult to follow. It is a reasonable, healthy way to eat, and it can be followed for an extended period of time.

If you are on the Carbohydrate-Sensitive Plan, continue to eat an unlimited amount of protein, but increase your carbohydrate intake to between 40 and 60 grams daily in Phase 2. In addition, you can still eat unlimited quantities of Free Foods and your one protein shake daily. (See Free Foods list on page 57 and protein shake recipe on page 59.)

If you are on the Calorie-Sensitive Plan, increase your total caloric intake to 1,600, mainly in the form of protein. That means bigger servings of meat, chicken, and fish. Continue to eat 60 grams of carbohydrates daily, along with unlimited quantities of Free Foods and your one protein shake daily. (See Free Foods list on page 57.)

You will lose weight at a slower pace. Don't worry, that's exactly what's supposed to happen. Expect to lose about two pounds of body fat the first few weeks and one pound every week thereafter. As long as you are steadily losing weight each week, stay on Phase 2 until you reach your desired weight.

PROBLEM: What If You Plateau?

If, after a few weeks or even months on Phase 2, you stop losing one pound a week before you reach your goal, you need to change what you are doing.

- If you are on the Carbohydrate-Sensitive Plan, switch over to Phase 1 of the Calorie-Sensitive Plan. If you don't start losing again, you need a Metabolic Tune-Up (see page 35). You will enjoy a month or two of eating normally until your metabolism is moving in the right direction. Once you have increased your metabolism, start on Phase 1 of the Calorie-Sensitive Plan.

- If you are on the Calorie-Sensitive Plan and you stop losing weight, you need a Metabolic Tune-Up (see page 35). After you have raised your metabolism, go back to Phase 1 and cycle through the program again.
- People who want to lose 50 or more pounds may have to cycle through the phases several times before they can achieve their desired goal, periodically stopping for a Metabolic Tune-Up.

PROBLEM: You Need a Break from Your Weight-Loss Program

People can get tired of dieting, especially if they have a great deal of weight to lose. If this happens to you, all isn't lost. Give yourself a Metabolic Tune-Up (see page 35). Think of it as a holding pattern. You can resume eating normally, but you won't gain any additional weight, and you won't lose any weight, either. You're giving yourself a time-out, free of fear, to regroup until you are reenergized and ready to resume your weight-loss efforts. When you are ready to go back on the meal plan, start over in Phase 1.

PROBLEM: What If You Fall Off the Diet?

There are distractions in life—good and bad—that may come between you and your weight-loss efforts. If you fall off the diet for a few days, a few weeks, or even a few months, just begin again when you are ready. Since the Curves Weight-Loss and Fitness Plan protects muscle as you burn fat, you are less likely to regain as much weight as you might have in the past on other diets. If you can maintain your workout even if you aren't watching your diet, you will still be ahead of the game.

How do you resume your diet? If you have more than 20 pounds to lose, start on Phase 1 for two weeks before moving to Phase 2. If you have less than 20 pounds to lose, start on Phase 1 for one week before moving to Phase 2.

And don't beat yourself up. As I tell my clients, two steps forward and one step backward will still get you to your destination.

Phase 3—Success!

GOAL: RESET YOUR METABOLISM SO YOU CAN LIBER-
ATE YOURSELF FROM PERPETUAL DIETING

HOW LONG: EAT NORMALLY AND HEALTHFULLY FOR A LIFE-
TIME OF A LEAN BODY AND GREAT HEALTH

Your commitment and hard work has paid off, and you have achieved your weight-loss goals. Now the challenge is to maintain your new body without living on a low-calorie diet. Phase 3 will raise your metabolic rate so that you can eat a normal amount of food without gaining weight.

On Phase 3, you will eat between 2,500 and 3,000 calories daily. That's a generous amount of food. You can stop counting carbohydrates and calories. Although I don't want you to monitor each morsel of food that goes into your mouth, it's a good idea to have some concept of what you should be putting on your plate. If you are clueless about nutrition, Chapter 7 will provide the basic information about how to eat well. But remember, you don't have to eat like an angel to stay out of diet hell. As you will see, Phase 3 has built-in safeguards that will prevent you from ballooning up.

There are three simple steps to Phase 3:

STEP 1: Establish Your Low and High Weight

Your current weight—that is, your post-diet weight before you go on to Phase 3—is your *low* weight. Weigh yourself every morning before breakfast. Start eating normally and healthfully. I'm warning you ahead of time that you are going to gain a little bit of weight, and it is part of the plan. So go ahead and eat and don't get freaked out when you step on the scale again. Within a day or two, you will notice a weight gain of about three to five pounds. The added weight is mostly water and between one-half and one pound of fat. This is your *high* weight. Keep track of your weight daily on the charts on page 319. Your goal is to stay within the range between your low weight and your high weight, and to not gain any more weight.

Please note that some of you may have monthly weight fluctuations due to your menstrual periods. Women who are prone to bloating may gain an additional three pounds a few days before the start of their menstrual cycles. If you know that you are prone to gain a few pounds every month before your period, simply subtract the extra monthly weight gain from your true high weight so you don't go back to Phase 1 needlessly. In other words, those extra "period pounds" don't count.

STEP 2: Don't Exceed Your High Weight

As soon as you hit your high weight, go back to Phase 1 to burn off the fat. On Phase 1, you will quickly lose the water and the fat, probably within a day. When you are back to your low weight, resume normal eating. Try not to stay on Phase 1 for more than 72 hours or you will stimulate the production of starvation hormones.

STEP 3: Keep Going

Weigh yourself daily. Whenever you reach your high weight, go back to Phase 1 to burn off the fat. Try not to stay on Phase 1 for more than three days—as soon as you reach your low weight, start eating normally again. You will notice that it will take a longer period of time to reach your high weight. The key is to never diet long enough to restimulate production of starvation hormones. Within two or three months, most women are able to eat normally for weeks at a time and must go back to Phase 1 for only one or two days a month to maintain their weight. If your metabolism is a bit slower, it may take longer. If you party for a week and continually exceed 2,500 to 3,000 calories daily, you will find that you have to go back on Phase 1 more often to burn off the extra pounds. When you resume eating normally and healthfully, you will soon be back on schedule.

The Metabolic Tune-Up

GOAL: **RAISE YOUR METABOLISM SO YOU CAN LOSE WEIGHT SUCCESSFULLY**

HOW LONG: **BETWEEN ONE AND THREE MONTHS, OR WHEN YOU CAN EAT NORMALLY WITHOUT GAINING WEIGHT**

Who needs a Metabolic Tune-Up? You do, if you can identify with any of the following problems:

1. Your metabolism is in the dumps due to years of low-calorie dieting, and you are not losing enough weight on Phase 1.
2. You've reached those frustrating plateaus on Phase 2.
3. You need a respite from your weight-loss plan.

Although the Metabolic Tune-Up is similar to Phase 3, there is one important difference. Phase 3 is designed to help you maintain your desired weight. The Metabolic Tune-Up is designed to repair years of damage inflicted on your metabolism by dieting.

The purpose of the Metabolic Tune-Up is not to lose weight. Trying to lose weight with a sluggish metabolism is counterproductive and will only weaken your metabolism further. You need to increase your metabolism, and dieting now will further depress it. At the end of the Metabolic Tune-Up, you will not have gained weight or lost weight. You will have raised your metabolic rate so that you can diet successfully.

The only way to increase your metabolism is to eat more food. So that's exactly what you're going to do. If you have already begun the program, by now you should have kicked the sugar habit, and you're probably eating better than you ever have in your life. Although you are no longer on any meal plan, take these good habits to the Metabolic Tune-Up. Eat normally and healthfully, about 2,500 to 3,000 calories per day. I don't expect you to eat like an angel, but try not to revert to your bad habits. You will stop dieting and begin eating normally and healthfully until your metabolism has recovered.

There are three simple steps to the Metabolic Tune-Up.

STEP 1: Establish Your Low and High Weights

Your current weight is your *low* weight. Record it on a chart on page 322. Weigh yourself every morning before breakfast. Start eating normally and healthfully, 2,500 to 3,000 calories per day. You may soon notice a weight gain of about three to five pounds, depending on body size. The added weight is mostly water and between one-half and one pound of fat. This is your *high* weight. Keep track of your weight daily on your chart. Your goal is to stay between your low weight and your high weight, and to not gain any more weight.

STEP 2: Don't Exceed Your High Weight

As soon as you hit your high weight, go to Phase 1 to burn off the fat. On Phase 1, you will quickly lose the water and the fat, probably within a day or two. *Try not to stay on Phase 1 for more than 72 hours.* Doing so would stimulate the production of starvation hormones, which would further depress your metabolism. When you are back to your low weight, resume normal eating.

STEP 3: Keep Going

Weigh yourself daily. Whenever you reach your high weight, go back to Phase 1 to burn off the fat. Do not stay on Phase 1 for more than three days. As soon as you reach your low weight, start eating normally and healthfully again. Don't assume that if you are taking weight off easily it means that it's time to go back on a weight-loss diet. If you start dieting now, you will quickly plateau and end up right back where you started.

How do you know when your metabolism is repaired? When you first start your Metabolic Tune-Up, you will notice that you are dieting more frequently than you are eating normally. As your metabolism becomes accustomed to more food, it will take longer and longer to gain those extra pounds back. You are ready to resume your weight-loss diet when you can eat normally for three to four weeks at a time without gaining weight and only need to go on Phase 1 for one or two days a month. If you are eating 2,500 calories a day and not gaining weight, you can assume that you have raised your metabolism to 2,500 calories.

When you have completed your Metabolic Tune-Up, if you have more than 20 pounds to lose, go back to Phase 1 for two weeks and then move on to Phase 2. If you have less than 20 pounds to lose, go to Phase 1 for one week, and then move on to Phase 2.

Curves Profile

ELIZABETH A.

LARGO, FLORIDA

I joined Curves on November 30, 2000. At the time, I was 22 years old and I weighed 265 pounds. That's not bad for a world heavyweight boxing champion, but on a young woman it was less than becoming. I had all the excuses and reasons in the world to be fat. "It's in my genes," I would say apologetically. "I already have a man," I would say, and gesture in the direction of my fiancé of five years as he put on his jacket to go to the store to buy me more ice cream. "At least I'm healthy," I would point out, hiding the inhalers and bottles of medication my doctors had prescribed.

Things began to unravel during my last year of college. In December, I went to the eye doctor for a routine exam. He found some swelling around my optic nerves and suggested that I see a neurologist. I asked for the worst-case scenario. He told me, "It's probably a benign condition, but it could be a brain tumor." I underwent months and months of medical tests. In the midst of all this, I was in my final term at college and student teaching ninth- and tenth-grade English. Then, late in February, the relationship that I had always counted on abruptly ended, to my immense surprise and pain. Despite my distress, I focused on finishing college and managed to graduate cum laude in May 2000. I wore a size 24 dress to graduation. I was also diagnosed with a condition called pseudo-tumor cerebri (not a brain tumor), which, I learned, was brought on by my being overweight. That still wasn't enough to motivate me to do something about it. I began teaching high school, and I met my future husband, Maher. Maher pushed me to find that beautiful thin person hiding behind all that flab. We started slowly. He would run with me and help me watch what I ate. When someone left a flier about Curves on his door, he suggested that I call. Finally, after a lot of prodding, I did.

Up until then, the major obstacles preventing me from working out at a gym were lack of commitment and fear of embarrassment. But at Curves, I faced neither. I worked out with women just like me. They weren't perfect, they weren't supermodels looking down their perfect noses at the fat girl—they were real honest-to-goodness people like me. It was as if we were all in this together. I worked hard at Curves, going regularly and watching what I ate. I kept repeating the mantra that I heard at Curves: "Nothing tastes as good as thin feels."

That following Christmas, when we visited my family, I was 100 pounds lighter. The compliments poured in, but nothing felt as good as the sense of accomplishment that I felt. Today I can fit my whole body into one leg of the pants I wore in college. I went from a size 24 to a size 8. And now I feel good when my husband and I go out together because I know I look good.

I still teach high school. I think the kids respect me more because I'm no longer overweight. It may not be right and it may not be fair, but the reality is that people do judge you by how you look. I'm sure that I missed out on jobs because of my size.

Curves has become a way of life and also has helped me to create a life. Having dealt with the infertility issues that oftentimes accompany obese women, I finally got pregnant after I dropped all that weight! I had my first baby on October 2, 2002, and I was even still working out at Curves on September 31. The doctor told me that because I was in such great shape, my pregnancy and delivery were amazingly easy. Five weeks to the day after giving birth, I was back at Curves. I'm back down to a size 10 already, and I know that I will be wearing a size 6 by my birthday in May.

CHAPTER 3

TEST YOUR METABOLISM

Which Meal Plan Is Right for You?

When I first began working as a nutritional and fitness counselor, I observed that some women did extremely well on a particular diet, while other women not only didn't lose weight, but actually gained weight on the same diet. I realized early on that not every metabolism is the same. After training thousands of women, I discovered that some do great on a high-protein diet, and some don't. That's why the Curves Weight-Loss and Fitness Program offers two different meal plans: the Carbohydrate-Sensitive Plan and the Calorie-Sensitive Plan. The Carbohydrate-Sensitive Plan allows you to eat unlimited amounts of protein and restricts some, but not all, carbohydrates. The Calorie-Sensitive Plan allows you to eat plenty of protein to protect your muscle, as well as more carbohydrates, but it limits calories. Both plans will yield spectacular results, and you'll find that you're never hungry.

Which meal plan is best for you? Take the following tests designed by the Institute of Nutritional Science, a San Diego–based health research group.

Is This You?
Symptoms of Carbohydrate Sensitivity

Carbohydrates include a wide variety of foods, ranging from fruits and vegetables to breads, grains, and pasta, to chips, cookies, and soda. What do these seemingly unrelated foods have in common? All carbohydrates are broken down into glucose or sugar in the body. Some carbohydrates—notably starches and highly sweetened foods and beverages—are metabolized much faster than others. These foods trigger a sudden rise in blood sugar, which, as I will explain, can cause both health and mood problems. In the wrong hands, they can be highly addictive.

Some people are more sensitive to the effects of carbohydrates than others. Are you strongly affected by carbohydrates? Read the following list of symptoms. If you regularly experience seven or more of the symptoms, you are carbohydrate-sensitive and should follow the Carbohydrate-Sensitive Plan. If your results are inconclusive, take the two tests on pages 41–42 to help you better identify the weight-loss method that will work best for you.

- Nervousness
- Irritability
- Fatigue and exhaustion
- Faintness, dizziness, cold sweats, shakiness, or weak spells
- Depression
- Drowsiness, especially after meals or in mid-morning
- Headaches
- Digestive disturbances for no apparent reason
- Forgetfulness
- Insomnia
- Needless worrying
- Mental confusion
- Rapid pulse, especially after eating certain foods
- Muscle pains
- Antisocial behavior

Overemotional crying spells
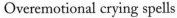 Lack of sex drive
Leg cramps and blurred vision
— Shortness of breath, sighing, and excessive yawning
✓ Cravings for starchy and sugar-rich foods

Test 1

Are You Carbohydrate-Sensitive?

Check yes or no for each of the eight statements below.

1. You are more than 25 pounds overweight.   *Yes* __X__   *No* ____

2. You have had a tendency to be overweight   *Yes* __X__   *No* ____
   for most of your life.

3. You have been overweight since you were   *Yes* __X__   *No* ____
   very young.

4. You have a poor appetite and often skip   *Yes* ____   *No* __X__
   meals.

5. You have food cravings that temporarily   *Yes* __✓__   *No* ____
   go away when you eat starchy or sugary
   foods.

6. You feel that there are foods that you   *Yes* __✓__   *No* ____
   absolutely could not live without.

7. Your waistline is bigger than your hips.   *Yes* ____   *No* __X__

8. At least five of the symptoms of   *Yes* __✓__   *No* ____
   carbohydrate sensitivity from the list
   above apply to you.

If you said yes to five or more of the statements in Test 1, you are likely to be carbohydrate-sensitive, and you should follow the Carbohydrate-Sensitive Meal Plan. If you did not check yes for five or more answers, take the following test.

Test 2
Are You Calorie-Sensitive?

Check yes or no for each of the eight statements below.

1. You didn't have a weight problem when you were younger, but you've slowly gained weight since turning 30.   Yes _____ No __X__

2. You are overweight by less than 25 pounds.   Yes _____ No __X__

3. You have a normal appetite and you get hungry at mealtimes.   Yes _____ No __X__

4. You have few, if any, food cravings.   Yes _____ No __X__

5. You have maintained the same basic eating habits all of your life.   Yes __X__ No _____

6. You eat three meals a day.   Yes __X__ No _____

7. You have gained weight in the past, but it seems to have tapered off (you are not continuing to gain steadily).   Yes _____ No __X__

8. You have less than five of the symptoms associated with poor carbohydrate metabolism (see list on pages 40–41).   Yes _____ No __X__

If you said yes to five or more of the statements in Test 2, you are likely to be calorie-sensitive and should follow the Calorie-Sensitive Meal Plan.

Still Not Sure?

By this point, most of you will know which plan you should follow. A small minority of you, however, may not yet have a conclusive answer. You may have answered yes to an equal number of questions in Test 1 and Test 2, and did not have five or more of the symptoms of carbohydrate sensitivity. If you fall into this group, start on the Carbohydrate-Sensitive Plan. If you don't lose at least three pounds in the first week and two pounds in the second week on the Carbohydrate-Sensitive Plan, switch to the Calorie-Sensitive Plan. If you can't lose weight on the Calorie-Sensitive Plan, you may need a Metabolic Tune-Up (see page 35). Your metabolism may have been so weakened by years of low-calorie and yo-yo dieting that it needs a period of recovery before you can successfully lose weight. When you go back on the meal plan, start with the Carbohydrate-Sensitive Plan, and if you don't lose at least three pounds in the first week and two pounds in the second week, switch to the Calorie-Sensitive Plan.

Now that you know which meal plan you should follow, let me tell you a bit more about the two Curves Meal Plans.

The Curves Meal Plans

- If you are carbohydrate-sensitive, you can eat unlimited amounts of protein and still lose weight if you cut back on starchy and sugary carbohydrates. As long as you are eating the right foods, your caloric intake doesn't matter. For you, the wrong carbohydrates can be addicting—the more you eat them, the more you want them. Your dependence on carbohydrates is harming your metabolism, locking you into fat-storage mode. Protein is the food that liberates you from carbohydrate slavery, freeing you to burn fat so you can finally stop dieting.

- If you are calorie-sensitive, you cannot lose weight if you eat unlimited amounts of protein, *even if you eliminate virtually all carbohydrates from your diet.* I bet many of you have been frustrated by the fact that when you go on popular all-you-can-eat high-protein diets, you tend to *gain* weight. In order for you to lose weight, you need to cut back on calories. This doesn't mean that excess carbohydrates are doing you any good. A high-carbohydrate diet is just as bad for you as it is for carbohydrate-sensitive people, although you may not show it in the same way. For one thing, eating lots of starchy carbohydrates will still cause the same sugar spikes that keep you constantly hungry—the last thing you need when you are counting calories. For another, if you don't eat enough protein, you will not maintain muscle or make new muscle. You need to eat enough protein to curb your hunger and keep your muscle cells pumping strongly. At the same time, you have to watch your calorie intake and maintain a strict limit, which you do in both Phase 1 and Phase 2.

Although there are significant differences between the two Curves Meal Plans, there are some important similarities, which I describe below.

More Protein

Both versions of the Curves Meal Plan are higher in protein than standard low-calorie weight-loss diets. Most of the popular low-calorie weight-loss diets recommend that women eat only about 11 percent of their daily calories from protein. On either version of the Curves Meal Plan, you will eat three to four times that amount in protein, and the pounds will still roll off you. The best part is that when you eat enough protein, you are more satisfied and not likely to get as hungry.

Down with Bad Carbohydrates

On either version of the Curves Meal Plan, you will limit your intake of starchy and sweet carbohydrates, such as bread, pasta, rice, and potatoes. Obviously, chips, cake, cookies, non-diet soda, and other junk food are off-limits entirely for people who need to lose weight. In Phase 2, you will be allowed to eat more starchy carbohydrates in the form of whole grains.

Up with Good Carbohydrates

Although high-protein diets tend to eliminate nearly all carbo-hydrates, especially in the first few weeks, the Curves Meal Plan allows you to fill up your plate with unlimited amounts of *healthy* carbo-hydrates, such as nonstarchy vegetables, that are burned more slowly and therefore do not cause dramatic swings in blood-sugar levels. Fruit is fine—up to a point. Although fruit is naturally high in sugar, it is also loaded with vitamins and other important disease-fighting chemicals. Some fruits, such as berries and melon, are lower in sugar than others and are therefore broken down more slowly in the body. We recommend that you stick to these low-sugar, low-carbohydrate fruits while you are on the Curves Meal Plan, and eat them in limited quantities. If you are on the Carbohydrate-Sensitive Plan, in Phase 1, when you are al-lowed only 20 grams of carbohydrates, fruit should be eaten rarely, if at all. In Phase 2, when you are allowed 60 grams of carbohydrates, you can have a daily serving of a low-sugar fruit if you like. (I provide a list of the carbohydrate content of commonly eaten fruits on pages 65–66.)

Problem Carbohydrates

You start your day off with a bagel, have a donut during your coffee break, grab a slice of pizza for lunch (the kind with the really thick crust), and snack on a frozen yogurt topped with fruit in the afternoon. By late afternoon, you're starving, and you reach for a candy bar to get you through until dinner. What's wrong with this picture?

You are consuming a steady diet of bad carbohydrates, and it is wreaking havoc on your metabolism. You are loading up on foods that are constantly flooding your body with glucose, or sugar. Your body re-acts to the sugar rush by producing insulin. As the insulin burns the sim-ple sugar off, it causes your blood sugar to drop too low, leaving you feeling ravenous and craving more carbohydrates. So you eat more starchy or sugary carbohydrates, and the same scenario is repeated over and over again throughout the day. You go up and down and up and down, and by late afternoon, you crash. (That's when you reach for the candy bar in your desk or hidden in the glove compartment of your car!)

Year after year of pumping too much insulin throughout your body desensitizes your body's tissues to insulin, which increases your risk of developing type II diabetes and other diseases of obesity, which I will discuss later.

If you are trying to lose weight, sugary carbohydrates will sabotage your efforts. When your body has a choice of burning a high-octane fuel like sugar or digging deep into your fat stores to burn fat, it will take the easy way out and burn sugar. If you don't give it a choice—if you cut back on sugary carbohydrates—it will be forced to burn fat. *If you want to switch from being a food-burning machine to being a fat-burning machine, you must reduce your intake of sugar-yielding starchy and sugary foods.*

If you are carbohydrate-sensitive, the sugar roller coaster can also put you in a really bad mood. As many of you know from firsthand experience, the sugar highs and lows will make you feel irritable, depressed, confused, and just plain lousy. When sugar levels drop precipitously, as they will if you are continually bombarding your body with sugar-yielding foods, you are placing your body under a great deal of stress. In fact, your body responds as if you are under attack and starts pumping stress hormones, also known as "flight or fight" hormones, throughout your body. These hormones in turn trigger a chain of reactions in which your body quite literally prepares for battle. That's why you often feel nervous or jittery when you are coming down from a sugar high. In order to calm down, you load up on more sugary foods, which is absolutely the worst thing that you can do. Relief is short-lived, and the cycle keeps repeating itself. Now do you understand why the wrong carbohydrates can sap your energy and cause you to quickly put on weight?

I'm not just talking about obvious junk carbohydrates like soda, chips, candy, and snack food. Even supposedly healthy foods, such as whole grains, bread, pasta, and even fruit, can be harmful in large quantities. Although they have more nutrients than outright junk food, they can still cause a steep rise in blood sugar, which will produce the sugar highs and lows in sensitive people.

I know that these foods are touted as beneficial by the medical establishment, and in fact, according to the U.S. government's food pyramid guide, we're supposed to eat up to 11 servings a day of starchy carbohydrates. That leaves room for only two to three small servings of protein daily. Why do the experts want you to fill up on sugar-yielding carbohydrates and not eat protein? It's not that they are so keen on carbohydrates, or that they have anything against protein—it's that they don't want you to eat too much fat. Since the 1980s, groups such as the American Heart Association and the American Dietetic Association have advised people to strictly limit their fat consumption because some forms of fat in the diet may boost cholesterol levels in the body, which in turn may increase the risk of developing heart disease. Unfortunately, protein has become a casualty of the fat debate. Protein happens to be a major source of fat in the diet, so reducing fat consumption in effect reduces protein intake.

The problem is, ever since these well-respected organizations issued this dietary advice, the obesity rate in the United States has doubled. Two decades ago, 30 percent of all Americans were overweight; now more than half are. There is no dispute that Americans are getting fatter. Why? Because if you don't eat fat or protein, what's left? Sugary carbohydrates!

I'm not advocating a high-fat diet, particularly if you are trying to lose weight, because fat is more calorie dense. But I think it's ridiculous not to eat protein because of a misguided "fat phobia." I recommend that you eat the leanest sources of protein with the least amount of saturated fat (the type of fat associated with an increased risk of heart disease in some people). On pages 60–62, you will see a list of the leanest and healthiest sources of protein, and I urge you to stick to this list as much as possible.

Insulin Resistance: The New Epidemic

Eating a diet high in sugar-yielding carbohydrates will not only hamper your ability to lose weight, but it may also increase your risk of developing serious metabolic diseases, such as insulin resistance and type II diabetes. There are two types of diabetes: type I (formerly called juvenile diabetes) and type II (also called adult-onset diabetes). Type I diabetes is caused by a failure of the pancreas to produce enough insulin to break down carbohydrates. Without adequate insulin, blood sugar can rise to dangerous levels, causing coma and even death. People with type I diabetes often require daily injections of insulin.

Type II diabetes is not caused by too little insulin—it is caused by too much insulin for too long. A disease that was once relatively rare and did not strike until late in life, type II diabetes is now becoming virtually epidemic in the United States among all age groups, even among children. With this condition, sufferers become insulin-resistant—that is, their pancreases are pumping out plenty of insulin, but their bodies do not utilize it efficiently. You can be mildly insulin-resistant for years before becoming diabetic. What causes insulin resistance? Insulin resistance occurs when your cells are constantly exposed to high levels of insulin. Eventually, your cells become immune to insulin's effect. What causes insulin levels to be chronically elevated? High-glucose-yielding carbohydrates! (These include pasta, potatoes, bagels, bread, fruit juice, candy, soda, etc.)

Insulin resistance can lead to serious health problems, including heart disease, high blood pressure, and blood-lipid abnormalities. It's interesting to note that these are exactly the conditions that a low-fat, high-carbohydrate diet was supposed to prevent.

The inability to use insulin effectively can have catastrophic effects on body composition. In other words, it can make you fat. Insulin not only controls blood sugar, it also operates the cellular machinery that accesses the energy in protein and fat. The same machinery determines whether the body will burn up its fat stores and make muscle or burn up its lean tissue—its muscle—and store fat. If you are insulin-resistant, you are stuck in fat-storage mode, and you will become flabby and overweight.

Between 1990 and 1998, there was a 70 percent increase in type II diabetes among adults between the ages of 30 and 39, and a 40 percent increase in adults between the ages of 40 and 49. Being overweight or obese puts you at greater risk of developing type II diabetes.

For obvious reasons, carbohydrate addicts are often insulin-resistant, and embarking on the Curves Carbohydrate-Sensitive Meal Plan is a great way to restore insulin sensitivity and prevent the downstream health problems. In addition, the Curves Workout will help make your cells more insulin-sensitive.

Pro Protein

If you want to liberate yourself from fat-storage mode, you must eat an adequate amount of protein. If you don't, you will be condemned to a very low-calorie diet for the rest of your life to maintain your weight loss. Protein is essential for several reasons:

- If you don't eat enough protein, you will lose too much muscle and will look flabby.
- Protein promotes thermogenesis—that is, it's a natural fat burner. People on a high-protein diet typically lose nearly twice as much weight as those on a high-carbohydrate weight-loss diet.
- Protein burns more slowly than carbohydrates, providing a steady stream of energy. It is more satisfying, and you won't get hungry as often if you eat more protein.

Carbohydrate-sensitive people have the added advantage of being able to eat unlimited amounts of protein and still lose weight. The obvious question is, how can you eat unlimited amounts of any food and not blow up? The answer is that a low-carbohydrate, high-protein diet forces your metabolism to shift gears, creating a situation in which calories become irrelevant. Here's what happens: Your brain uses glucose (sugar) as a primary energy source, and if you are not eating glucose-yielding foods (carbohydrates), your body will find another fuel source—fat. *Thus, your body stops storing fat and begins burning it up.* But what about all those extra protein calories? Why aren't they stored as fat? Remember, it takes insulin to store fat, and in a low-carbohydrate environment, your body is not producing very much insulin. Since many carbohydrate-sensitive people are somewhat insulin-resistant to begin with, the insulin that you are producing comes in way below the cellular radar. Your cells simply don't notice it. That's why people on high-protein, very low-carbohydrate diets are able to lose weight very rapidly, although they are still eating a lot of food.

The question is, are high-protein diets safe? When fat is burned as fuel, it produces by-products called ketones. Ketones build up in the body and are eventually eliminated through urine (via the kidneys), sweat, or breath. This might force your kidneys to work harder. If you do not have a kidney problem and are otherwise healthy, mild ketosis is harmless, as long as you drink enough water to flush out the ketones from the kidneys (at least eight glasses daily).

In most cases, you must eat 60 grams or less of carbohydrates daily to cause ketosis. On the Curves Meal Plan, you are usually in true ketosis for only one or two weeks. In Phase 2, you are allowed to consume 40 to 60 grams of carbohydrate, but you are actually eating a lot more, because that total does not include Free Foods, all of which contain carbohydrates, as well as your protein shake, which has 20 grams of carbohydrates. Nevertheless, you will continue to burn fat and lose weight since you are not consuming huge quantities of glucose-yielding carbohydrates.

Some studies have shown that high-protein diets can interfere with the absorption of calcium, which can promote osteoporosis, a bone-thinning disease. While you are on a high-protein diet, I recommend that you take a calcium supplement every day.

If you have liver or kidney problems, or are diabetic, you should talk to your doctor before going on any weight-loss diet, especially one that is high in protein and low in carbohydrates. A diet that induces ketosis is not recommended during pregnancy.

The only caveat is, you absolutely cannot cheat on the Carbohydrate-Sensitive Plan. I mean it—you can't cheat. You can only eat glucose-yielding carbohydrates in the right quantities or you will gain weight, not lose weight. Once you start eating excess carbohydrates, you will start producing more insulin, and those protein calories will begin to add up. Otherwise, a high-protein, low-carbohydrate diet is a terrific way to shed excess fat, and you won't be hungry all the time.

If a high-protein, low-carbohydrate diet is so great, why don't I recommend it for everyone? Calorie-sensitive people will not lose weight eating unlimited amounts of protein. Why? Their bodies are able to access the energy in protein and fat even in the absence of carbohydrates. Their cells are still sensitive to insulin, and it doesn't take very much of this hormone to keep them locked in fat-storage mode. That means that even if they eat minuscule quantities of glucose-producing foods, their bodies are able to burn the fat and protein in food, and do not have to dig into their fat stores. Therefore, if they eat more protein calories than they can burn, they will just store it as more fat. And since they are not burning up their fat stores, they will end up with more fat than they started out with. The only way calorie-sensitive people can become fat-burning machines is to eat fewer calories than they burn, but they should never starve themselves. Undereating can create even worse problems for these people than overeating, as you will see in Chapter 6. Calorie-sensitive people do best on a moderately high-protein diet that conforms to their calorie guidelines, with ample good carbohydrates.

Now that you understand which version of the Curves Meal Plan will work best for you, you are ready to start the program. In Part Two, you will see how the Curves Weight-Loss and Fitness Program will free you from a lifetime of dieting.

Curves Profile

APRIL N.

HAZELHURST, MISSISSIPPI

When I first joined Curves almost two years ago, I was 15 years old, weighed 272 pounds, and wore a size 28. Today, I wear a size 10 and have lost well over 100 pounds. My weight has been a constant struggle for my entire life. Being overweight runs in my family, and I just like to eat. My doctor finally told me that I had to do something about my weight because I was putting my health at risk. I tried several different diets, but they didn't work for me, and I even took a prescription diet pill. I lost 20 pounds on the diet pills, but when I stopped taking them, I regained 50 pounds. I tried everything, and then one day I finally decided to get serious about it. I knew the only way to lose weight was to exercise and to eat right. It's a lifestyle choice. You can't blame your parents and you can't blame your genes—it's up to you. So I joined Curves.

When I first started on the Curves: Permanent Results Without Permanent Dieting program, no one thought it would work, because I had tried so many other diets before. I started doing the exercise program three times a week, and I began following the Carbohydrate-Sensitive Meal Plan (the low-carb program). Much to everyone's surprise—including my own—the weight began to come off of me, a lot at first and then at a steady pace. I kept with it, and I finally reached my goal.

Everybody is amazed at how I've changed. I'm pretty amazed about it myself. My friends are very supportive. I don't eat pasta or pizza, and I don't eat a lot of bread, and when we go out to dinner, my friends make sure that we always go someplace where I can eat some protein and a big salad. I eat a much healthier diet than I used to. I never want to gain the weight back, and my friends don't want me to gain the weight back either.

My life has changed a lot since I've lost all that weight. I used to hate to buy clothes; now I love it. It's fun. I even like buying bathing suits! I spent the last two summers working as a lifeguard. I felt *great* in my bathing suit. Before I started Curves, I wanted to be a lawyer. Now I'm planning on going to college to major in exercise science, because I want to devote my life to helping other overweight people lose weight. I work as a trainer at Curves after school. I really like encouraging people who have a weight problem. I tell them to just stick with it because, if they do, the program will work. I show them my before picture, and they can see what I look like now. I always tell them, "If I can do it, you can do it."

PART TWO

The Curves

Weight-Loss and

Fitness Program

KEEPING TRACK OF CALORIES AND CARBOHYDRATES

A List of Common Foods

On the food lists that follow, you will see a wide selection of food choices to help you succeed on the Curves Meal Plan. Try to plan your daily meals around these foods. In Chapter 5, The Carbohydrate-Sensitive Plan, and Chapter 6, The Calorie-Sensitive Plan, I provide sample menus for each of the two phases of the meal plans. You can follow my suggested menus, or you can use my menus as a guide to put together meals of your own, based on your likes and dislikes.

I have provided blank meal-planning pages in your Daily Meal Planner, and you can download additional pages off my website, www.curvesinternational.com.

Free Foods

Whether you are following the Carbohydrate-Sensitive Plan or the Calorie-Sensitive Plan, you can eat as much of these Free Foods as you want. You should not include them in your calorie or carbohydrate count.

Alfalfa sprouts
Arugula

Asparagus
Bamboo shoots
Bean sprouts (cooked or canned)
Bibb lettuce
Bok choy
Broccoli
Brussels sprouts
Cabbage, red and green
Cauliflower
Celery
Cilantro
Cucumbers
Dill pickles
Endive
Garlic
Kale
Kohlrabi
Mushrooms
Mustard greens
Onions (not sweet)
Parsley
Peppers, red, green, yellow, and orange
Radishes
Romaine lettuce
Sauerkraut
Scallions
Snow peas
Spinach
Summer squash
Watercress
Zucchini

FREE FLAVORINGS
Lemon juice
Yellow mustard

Free for All!
Your Protein Shake

One of your six meals each day can be a high-protein shake, which, if you prepare it correctly, can taste like a terrific milk shake. (No kidding, really!) Even better, the basic shake is a *Free Food*, so it doesn't count in your calorie or carbohydrate total. We have our own Curves Shake, which is a soy-based protein shake that comes in vanilla and chocolate flavors, but there are also other brands of protein shakes on the market that you can use. Be sure to buy a brand that contains at least 20 grams of protein and no more than 20 grams of carbohydrates. Please try to find a brand that is low in sugar or at least does not contain sucrose (table sugar). We sweeten our shake with stevia, a natural sweetener that is very low in calories, and a touch of fructose (fruit sugar). Some protein powders contain artificial sweeteners. Beware of premade protein shakes! Some so-called protein shakes are no more than highly sugared, watered-down milk. You can buy flavored protein powder or unflavored protein powder at most health-food stores, some supermarkets, and even at warehouse stores and discount general-merchandise stores. Protein powder can be mixed with water or skim milk. For a frothy texture, mix the shake in a blender with 4 or 5 ice cubes. For variety, add a teaspoon of vanilla extract (10 calories and 1 carbohydrate gram) or a teaspoon of pure almond extract (11 calories) or ½ teaspoon of orange extract (11 calories). You can also add ¼ cup of fresh berries for flavoring, but you must count the berries in your carbohydrate total for the day.

	grams of carbohydrate	calories
Protein		
Poultry		
4-oz. chicken breast, no skin	0	124
1 chicken sausage	3	100
1 chicken hot dog	3	120
4 oz. fajita chicken	0	120
½ Cornish hen, no skin	0	150
4-oz. turkey breast, no skin	0	120
4 oz. deli turkey breast	4	120
4-oz. ground turkey patty	0	176
2 strips turkey bacon	0	70
1 turkey hot dog	4	120
2.5 oz. turkey breakfast sausages (about 3 links)	2	120
Beef and Veal		
4-oz. beef tenderloin	0	244
3.5-oz. flank steak	0	224
4-oz. sirloin steak	0	215
4 oz. roast beef, deli	4	120
4-oz. hamburger patty (93% lean)	0	160
4-oz. hamburger patty (96% lean)	0	130
3.5-oz. veal loin chop	0	284
Pork		
4-oz. center-cut pork chop, lean	0	150
4-oz. pork loin	0	150
3 oz. lean ham	0	120
4 oz. smoked sausage, low-fat	8	220
1 link breakfast sausage, low-fat	0	67

	grams of carbohydrate	calories
Pork *(continued)*		
3 strips bacon, pan-broiled	0	110
2 strips Canadian bacon, pan-broiled	0	87
Lamb		
3.5 oz. leg of lamb	0	180
3.5-oz. loin chop	0	320
3.5 oz. shoulder, for stew	0	225
Game		
4 oz. venison, roasted	0	180
6-oz. buffalo burger	0	300
Fish and Seafood		
6 oz. bass	0	200
6 oz. cod	0	140
6 oz. flounder	0	160
6 oz. haddock	0	150
6 oz. halibut	0	240
3 oz. mackerel	0	175
6 oz. orange roughy	0	162
6 oz. perch	0	150
6 oz. pike	0	150
6 oz. pollack	0	200
6 oz. rainbow trout	0	280
3 oz. salmon	0	155
4.25 oz. sardines (one can, in oil)	2	190
8 oz. shrimp	0	240
7 oz. scallops	4	175
6 oz. snapper	0	170

	grams of carbohydrate	calories
Fish and Seafood *(continued)*		
2.8 oz. tuna (one small can, in water)	0	100
6 oz. tuna, fresh	0	185
6 oz. turbot	0	160
Eggs		
1 large	1	75
Tofu		
3 oz. (extra-firm)	1	90

Dairy Products

Milk

	grams of carbohydrate	calories
8 oz. skim	12	84
8 oz. 2% fat	12	120
8 oz. whole	12	150
2 Tbsp. half-and-half	0	35
1 Tbsp. whipping cream	0	52

Yogurt

	grams of carbohydrate	calories
8 oz. plain, low-fat	18	150

Soft Cheeses

	grams of carbohydrate	calories
1 oz. Brie	0	95
1 oz. Camembert	0	85
½ cup cottage cheese (1% fat)	5	80
½ cup cottage cheese (2% fat)	5	90
2 Tbsp. cream cheese	1	100

	grams of carbohydrate	calories
Soft Cheeses *(continued)*		
2 Tbsp. light cream cheese	1	74
2 Tbsp. vegetable cream cheese	2	90
¼ cup ricotta	3	110
Semisoft Cheeses		
1 oz. (2 Tbsp.) blue, crumbled	0	95
1 oz. brick	0	110
1 oz. feta	0	80
1 Tbsp. feta, reduced fat, crumbled	0	15
1 oz. Havarti	0	120
1 oz. Monterey Jack	0	110
1 oz. Muenster	0	100
1 oz. pepper jack	0	110
1 oz. provolone	0	100
Hard Cheeses		
1 oz. cheddar	0	110
1 oz. Colby	0	110
1 oz. Edam	0	90
1 oz. Gouda	0	110
1 oz. Swiss	0	110
Very Hard Cheeses		
1 Tbsp. grated Parmesan	0	28
¼ cup shredded Parmesan	0	110
1 Tbsp. grated Romano	0	28

	grams of carbohydrate	calories
Other		
1 slice (¾ oz.) American Pasteurized Processed Cheese Food	0	80

Grains and Starches

	grams of carbohydrate	calories
1 Tbsp. all-purpose flour	7	28
1 Tbsp. cornstarch	7	30
½ cup refried beans, traditional	25	120
1 piece Holland rusk dry toast	6	30
1 slice Pepperidge Farm light bread	9	45
1 slice whole-wheat bread	12	70
2 Tbsp. All-Bran Cereal	6	20
1 cup oatmeal, cooked, old-fashioned	27	150
2 RyKrisp crackers	11	60
2 Keebler Harvest Bakery Multigrain Crackers	11	70
2 Kavi crackers	15	70
3 slices Devonsheer melba toast	11	50
1 cup cooked long-grain brown rice	45	216
1 cup cooked long-grain white rice	45	205
1 cup cooked spaghetti	40	197
1 medium white baked potato with skin	51	220
½ cup cooked yam	19	79

Miscellaneous

	grams of carbohydrate	calories
1 cup beef broth, canned	0	18
1 cup chicken broth, canned	1	30
½ cup chocolate chips	52	440
2 Tbsp. chocolate syrup	24	100

	grams of carbohydrate	calories
Miscellaneous *(continued)*		
1 oz. unsweetened chocolate	4	95
½ cup chocolate ice cream	19	160
½ cup French vanilla ice cream	15	160
½ cup brandy	0	296
½ cup white or rosé wine	6	120
½ cup red wine	0	88
2 Tbsp. dry sherry	5	35
1 Tbsp. brown sugar, packed	13	51
1 Tbsp. white sugar	12	46
Condiments		
1 Tbsp. barbeque sauce	6	25
1 Tbsp. Heinz 57 sauce	5	18
2 Tbsp. salsa	2	10
1 Tbsp. soy sauce	1	10
¼ tsp. Tabasco sauce	0	0
1 Tbsp. wine vinegar	1	2
1 tsp. Worcestershire sauce	1	5
½ Tbsp. yellow mustard	0	1
1 Tbsp. Heinz tomato ketchup	6	15
1 Tbsp. A1 steak sauce	3	15
1 Tbsp. Lea & Perrins Traditional Steak Sauce	6	25
Fruits		
1 small apple, with peel	20	80
½ medium banana	13	53
¼ cup blueberries	7	27

	grams of carbohydrate	calories
Fruits *(continued)*		
½ cup cantaloupe, cubed	6	25
⅓ cup cranberries, dried and sweetened	33	130
½ medium grapefruit	12	46
½ cup grapes, seedless	14	57
1½ Tbsp. lime juice	1	5
1 medium nectarine	16	67
1 medium orange	16	65
2½ Tbsp. fresh orange juice	4	17
8 oz. orange juice, from concentrate	28	110
8 oz. orange juice, fresh	26	112
1 medium peach, peeled	9	37
1 medium plum	9	36
¼ cup raspberries	4	17
½ cup strawberries	6	23
½ cup watermelon, cubed	6	25
1 medium tomato	5.7	26
Nuts		
1 oz. almonds, roasted and salted	4	180
1 oz. cashews, roasted and salted	7	170
1 oz. macadamia nuts, roasted and salted	5	160
1 oz. peanuts	5	160
2 oz. pistachios, in shells	7	170
2 Tbsp. soy nuts, honey-roasted	5	58
1 Tbsp. sunflower seed kernels, roasted and salted	1	47
1 oz. walnuts, shelled	4	190
1 oz. dry-roasted pecans, salted	6.3	187

Free Foods Salad

On the sample menus in the following chapters, you will see references to the Free Foods Salad. It's easy to make. Just cut up any (or all) of the vegetables on the Free Foods list (see page 57) into bite-size pieces and put them in a salad bowl. Dress with a tablespoon of your favorite low-calorie dressing (no more than 4 grams of carbohydrates and 50 calories per two tablespoons) or a tablespoon of olive oil with a bit of lemon juice. (Who says there's no such thing as a free lunch?) Add a protein portion to your salad, and you have a quick and easy meal.

CURVES TIP: COOKING FOR YOUR FAMILY · Many of you have the responsibility of cooking for your family as well as for yourself, and the fact that you are on a diet isn't going to change that. The menus that I provide can be adapted quite nicely for your family by adding an extra starch (potato, rice, or pasta) or fruit with the meal. Of course, non-dieting family members can eat larger portions and don't have to worry about counting their calories or carbohydrates. Everyone in the family, however, will benefit from eating more lean protein, lots of high-fiber vegetables, and less overly processed, nutrient-poor food. If members of your family eat dessert or indulge in snack foods, ask them to do so out of your sight if you find these foods hard to resist.

Curves Profile

JAYME P.

COLORADO SPRINGS, COLORADO

I have battled with my weight forever. Ten years ago, when I weighed 275 pounds and was in a terrible marriage, I went on a crazy starvation diet. I saw a diet doctor, who gave me metabolism-booster shots. It was a nightmare—I lost 100 pounds in less than a year, and now that I think about it, it's pretty amazing that I didn't have a heart attack or a stroke. Then I got divorced and gained back almost all my weight. I had been divorced for nearly six years and weighed close to 230 pounds when my mom and my sister told me that they were going to open a Curves. They wanted me to join! I thought they were crazy—I had never exercised before. I had always been the overweight, sedentary one in the family—that's just who I was—and I thought I would always be that way. They opened their first location in January 1999. They begged me to come in and try it, and I finally gave in.

I tried it, and in the first month—*without dieting*—just doing the Curves circuit, I lost eight inches and four pounds. I thought, *Wow, I can do this!* And so I kept doing it. Then I began to follow the Curves Meal Plan. Phase 3 has been my savior. Phase 3 is why I've been able to keep the weight off for two years. I still have moments—especially on the weekends—when I binge eat. Phase 3 saves me because when I get on that scale on Monday morning and I see those three pounds, I know it's time to go back to Phase 1 for a couple of days, and I knock them right back off. Losing 135 pounds over a lifetime is a big deal. I know that. But it's not half as big a deal as keeping it off. *Keeping it off is a big deal.*

I got remarried last year. I wore a size 8 wedding dress. By the way, I started dating my current husband when I was 55 pounds heavier than I am right now. So he has gone through the experience of me losing all this weight and changing my life, and he has been very supportive.

It really is a lifestyle change. You have to accept that you must exercise to be strong, maintain muscle, and keep excess weight off. You do have to pay attention to the scale, and so it affects your whole life, but in a very positive way.

The secret is, it's really not that hard to do. It's 30 minutes of exercise. I mean, hello, it's *30 minutes*. For the most part, you can eat all day long, as long as you eat the right things. For overweight people, we don't think about eating the right thing very often or we wouldn't be overweight to begin with. At first it's very difficult, I think, but once you decide to do it, you just make the change.

I wouldn't have ever believed it could happen, but I now work as a fitness manager at a Curves. This year, from Thanksgiving through New Year's, I ran a special Phase 3 class. It helps women enjoy the holidays and partake in holiday meals without adding extra weight. For some women, it's exactly what they need.

I am convinced that Curves is a God-given solution for overweight women everywhere.

CHAPTER 5

THE CARBOHYDRATE-SENSITIVE PLAN

I n the pages that follow, you will find seven weeks of sample menus on the Carbohydrate-Sensitive Plan: two weeks of Phase 1 menus and five weeks of Phase 2 menus. You can follow these menus or you can change the order of the meals as you see fit. You may find that you like some meals but dislike others. Use the blank menu forms on pages 311–16 in your Daily Meal Planner to customize the meal plan to reflect your tastes. As long as you stay within your carbohydrate guidelines, you can be as creative as you like.

In the Daily Meal Planner, you will also find weekly shopping lists for these menus, and recipes for the special Curves meals listed in the menus. Please note that the ingredients for the special recipes are not included in the weekly shopping lists, for the simple reason that not everyone likes to cook. If you choose to make these dishes, you must add the ingredients to your weekly shopping list.

Count your carbohydrates for each meal and record the total on your Daily Meal Planner. (If you use the sample menus, we've done the counting for you.)

Phase 1

- If you want to lose less than 20 pounds, follow Phase 1 for only one week.
- If you want to lose more than 20 pounds, stay on Phase 1 for two weeks.
- At the end of Phase 1, move on to Phase 2.

You can eat unlimited amounts of protein (including lean meats, cheeses, eggs, seafood, and poultry) but *no more than 20 grams of carbohydrates*. In addition, you are allowed unlimited amounts of Free Foods and your one protein shake daily. If you are on the Carbohydrate-Sensitive Plan, you must drink at least eight glasses of water daily.

PROBLEM: What If You Don't Lose Enough?
Although most women will lose a substantial amount of weight on Phase 1 (between 6 and 10 pounds), a small minority may not.

- If you have not lost at least three pounds the first week, and have lost less than two pounds the second week, switch to the Calorie-Sensitive Plan. If within a week you still haven't lost at least three pounds, go to the Metabolic Tune-Up for a metabolic adjustment (see page 35).

Phase 2

Stay on Phase 2 until you reach your desired weight, you plateau, or you want a break from dieting.

During Phase 2, you eat more food and a greater variety of food. You should lose one to two pounds per week. Continue to eat an unlimited amount of protein, but increase your carbohydrate intake to between 40 and 60 grams daily. In addition, you can still eat unlimited quantities of Free Foods and your one protein shake daily.

As long as you are steadily losing weight, stay on Phase 2 until you reach your desired weight.

PROBLEM: What If You Plateau?

If after a few weeks or even months on Phase 2, you stop losing one pound a week before you reach your goal, you need to change what you are doing.

- Switch to the Calorie-Sensitive Plan (see page 100), starting with Phase 1. If you don't start losing weight again, you need a Metabolic Tune-Up (see page 35). It could take one to three months to get your metabolism high enough to begin losing again. Once you have raised your metabolism, start again on Phase 1 of the Calorie-Sensitive Program.
- People who want to lose 50 or more pounds may have to cycle through the phases several times before they can achieve their desired goal, periodically stopping for a Metabolic Tune-Up (see page 35).

PROBLEM: What If You Want Time Off?

If you need some time off from your weight-loss plan, give yourself a Metabolic Tune-Up (see page 35). When you are ready to resume your weight-loss regimen, go back to Phase 1.

KEEPING TRACK · Count your calories and carbohydrates for each meal, and record the total on your Daily Meal Planner (see page 311).

Phase 1
Week 1
Monday

		Carbs	Calories
Meal 1	½ cup strawberries	6	23
	½ cup cottage cheese, 1% fat	5	80
Meal 2	1 Curves Shake or similar protein shake (see page 59)	FREE	FREE
Meal 3	1 Free Foods Salad	FREE	FREE
	6 oz. ground beef, 93% lean, broiled	0	240
Meal 4	2 stalks celery	FREE	FREE
	2 Tbsp. vegetable cream cheese	2	90
Meal 5	1 serving Parmesan Vegetable Stir-Fry (see page 304)	0	175
	6-oz. chicken breast, broiled	0	186
Meal 6	3 oz. ham, lean	0	120

Week 1
Tuesday

Meal 1	4 strips bacon	0	147
	1 egg	1	75
Meal 2	½ cup cantaloupe, cubed	6	25
	½ cup cottage cheese, 1% fat	5	80
Meal 3	1 Free Foods Salad	FREE	FREE
	4 oz. turkey breast, deli	4	120
Meal 4	1 Curves Shake or similar protein shake (see page 59)	FREE	FREE
Meal 5	½ cup broccoli, steamed	FREE	FREE
	½ cup cauliflower, steamed	FREE	FREE
	1 Tbsp. butter	0	102
	6 oz. sirloin steak, broiled	0	323
Meal 6	1 oz. Havarti cheese	0	120

Week 1 Wednesday		Carbs	Calories
Meal 1	4 oz. yogurt, plain	9	75
Meal 2	1 Curves Shake or similar protein shake (see page 59)	FREE	FREE
Meal 3	1 Free Foods Salad	FREE	FREE
	4 oz. roast beef, deli	4	120
Meal 4	1 serving Tuna Salad (see page 295)	3	258
Meal 5	½ cup zucchini sauteed in	FREE	FREE
	½ Tbsp. olive oil	0	60
	6-oz. pork chop, lean, broiled	0	225
Meal 6	1 medium dill pickle	FREE	FREE
	3 oz. ham, lean	0	120
	1 oz. cheddar cheese	0	110

Week 1 Thursday			
Meal 1	2 sausage links	0	134
	2 eggs	2	150
Meal 2	½ cup baby carrots	5	24
	½ cup cottage cheese, 1% fat	5	80
Meal 3	1 Free Foods Salad	FREE	FREE
	2.8 oz. (one small can) tuna, in water	0	100
Meal 4	1 Curves Shake or similar protein shake (see page 59)	FREE	FREE
Meal 5	1 serving Chicken Fajitas (see page 293)	1	280
Meal 6	2 oz. Havarti cheese	0	240

Week 1 Friday

Meal		Carbs	Calories
Meal 1	3 oz. ham, lean	0	120
	2 eggs	2	150
Meal 2	½ cup cantaloupe, cubed	6	25
	½ cup cottage cheese, 1% fat	5	80
Meal 3	½ cup brussels sprouts, steamed	FREE	FREE
	1 tsp. butter	0	34
	6 oz. salmon, broiled	0	310
Meal 4	1 Curves Shake or similar protein shake (see page 59)	FREE	FREE
Meal 5	1 Free Foods Salad	FREE	FREE
	4 oz. turkey bacon	0	160
Meal 6	2 stalks celery	FREE	FREE
	1 oz. cheddar cheese	0	110

Week 1 Saturday

Meal		Carbs	Calories
Meal 1	3 sausage links	0	200
	2 eggs	2	150
Meal 2	1 Curves Shake or similar protein shake (see page 59)	FREE	FREE
Meal 3	1 Free Foods Salad	FREE	FREE
	8 oz. cooked salad shrimp	0	240
Meal 4	1 medium dill pickle	FREE	FREE
	4 oz. ground beef, 93% lean, broiled	0	160
Meal 5	1 serving French Onion Soup (see page 290)	3	145
	8-oz. cod fillet, broiled	0	186
Meal 6	4 oz. yogurt, plain	9	75

Week 1 Sunday		Carbs	Calories
Meal 1	3 sausage links	0	200
	2 eggs	2	150
Meal 2	1 cup asparagus, steamed	FREE	FREE
	½ Tbsp. butter	0	51
	4 oz. chicken breast, broiled	0	124
Meal 3	1 Free Foods Salad	FREE	FREE
Meal 4	½ cup cantaloupe, cubed	6	25
	½ cup cottage cheese, 1% fat	5	80
Meal 5	½ cup cauliflower, steamed	FREE	FREE
	1 cup spinach	FREE	FREE
	8 oz. orange roughy, sauteed in	0	216
	1 Tbsp. olive oil	0	120
Meal 6	1 Curves Shake or similar protein shake (see page 59)	FREE	FREE

Week 2 Monday			
Meal 1	½ cup strawberries	6	23
	½ cup cottage cheese, 1% fat	5	80
Meal 2	1 Curves Shake or similar protein shake (see page 59)	FREE	FREE
Meal 3	1 Free Foods Salad	FREE	FREE
	6 oz. ground beef, 93% lean, broiled	0	240
Meal 4	2 stalks celery	FREE	FREE
	2 Tbsp. vegetable cream cheese	2	90
Meal 5	1 serving Parmesan Vegetable Stir-Fry (see page 304)	0	175
	6 oz. chicken breast, broiled	0	186
Meal 6	3 oz. ham, lean	0	120

Week 2 Tuesday

Meal		Carbs	Calories
Meal 1	4 strips bacon	0	147
	1 egg	1	75
Meal 2	½ cup cantaloupe, cubed	6	25
	½ cup cottage cheese, 1% fat	5	80
Meal 3	1 Free Foods Salad	FREE	FREE
	4 oz. turkey breast, deli	4	120
Meal 4	1 Curves Shake or similar protein shake (see page 59)	FREE	FREE
Meal 5	½ cup broccoli, steamed	FREE	FREE
	½ cup cauliflower, steamed	FREE	FREE
	1 Tbsp. butter	0	102
	6 oz. sirloin steak, broiled	0	323
Meal 6	1 oz. Havarti cheese	0	120

Week 2 Wednesday

Meal		Carbs	Calories
Meal 1	4 oz. yogurt, plain	9	75
Meal 2	1 Curves Shake or similar protein shake (see page 59)	FREE	FREE
Meal 3	1 Free Foods Salad	FREE	FREE
	4 oz. roast beef, deli	4	120
Meal 4	1 serving Tuna Salad (see page 295)	3	258
Meal 5	½ cup zucchini, sauteed in	FREE	FREE
	½ Tbsp. olive oil	0	60
	6-oz. pork chop, lean, broiled	0	225
Meal 6	1 medium dill pickle	FREE	FREE
	3 oz. ham, lean	0	120
	1 oz. cheddar cheese	0	110

Week 2 Thursday

		Carbs	Calories
Meal 1	2 sausage links	0	134
	2 eggs	2	150
Meal 2	½ cup baby carrots	5	24
	½ cup cottage cheese, 1% fat	5	80
Meal 3	1 Free Foods Salad	FREE	FREE
	2.8 oz. (one small can) tuna, in water	0	100
Meal 4	1 Curves Shake or similar protein shake (see page 59)	FREE	FREE
Meal 5	1 serving Chicken Fajitas (see page 293)	1	280
Meal 6	2 oz. Havarti cheese	0	240

Week 2 Friday

		Carbs	Calories
Meal 1	3 oz. ham, lean	0	120
	2 eggs	2	150
Meal 2	½ cup cantaloupe, cubed	6	25
	½ cup cottage cheese, 1% fat	5	80
Meal 3	½ cup brussels sprouts, steamed	FREE	FREE
	1 tsp. butter	0	34
	6 oz. salmon, broiled	0	310
Meal 4	1 Curves Shake or similar protein shake (see page 59)	FREE	FREE
Meal 5	1 Free Foods Salad	FREE	FREE
	4 oz. turkey bacon	0	160
Meal 6	2 stalks celery	FREE	FREE
	1 oz. cheddar cheese	0	110

Week 2 Saturday

Meal		Carbs	Calories
Meal 1	3 sausage links	0	200
	2 eggs	2	150
Meal 2	1 Curves Shake or similar protein shake (see page 59)	FREE	FREE
Meal 3	1 Free Foods Salad	FREE	FREE
	8 oz. cooked salad shrimp	0	240
Meal 4	1 medium dill pickle	FREE	FREE
	6 oz. ground beef, 93% lean, broiled	0	240
Meal 5	8 oz. cod fillet, broiled	0	186
	1 serving French Onion Soup (see page 290)	3	145
Meal 6	4 oz. yogurt, plain	9	75

Week 2 Sunday

Meal		Carbs	Calories
Meal 1	3 sausage links	0	200
	2 eggs	2	150
Meal 2	1 cup asparagus, steamed	FREE	FREE
	½ Tbsp. butter	0	51
	6-oz. chicken breast, broiled	0	186
Meal 3	1 Free Foods Salad	FREE	FREE
Meal 4	½ cup cantaloupe, cubed	6	25
	½ cup cottage cheese, 1% fat	5	80
Meal 5	½ cup cauliflower, steamed	FREE	FREE
	1 tsp. butter	0	34
	1 cup spinach	FREE	FREE
	8 oz. orange roughy, sauteed in	0	216
	1 Tbsp. olive oil	0	120
Meal 6	1 Curves Shake or similar protein shake (see page 59)	FREE	FREE

		Carbs	Calories
Phase 2 Week 1 Monday			
Meal 1	½ cup strawberries	6	23
	½ cup cottage cheese, 1% fat	5	80
Meal 2	1 Curves Shake or similar protein shake (see page 59)	FREE	FREE
Meal 3	1 Free Foods Salad	FREE	FREE
	1 serving French Onion Soup (see page 290)	3	145
	6 oz. ground beef, 93% lean, broiled	0	240
Meal 4	2 RyKrisp crackers	11	60
	1 serving Tuna Salad (see page 295)	3	258
Meal 5	1 serving Chinese Vegetables (see page 303)	8	160
	6-oz. chicken breast, broiled	0	186
	1 serving Italian Soda (see page 307)	0	100
Meal 6	2 oz. ham, lean	0	80
	1 oz. Havarti cheese	0	120
	1 peach, medium	9	37
Week 1 Tuesday			
Meal 1	1 tomato, sliced	5.7	26
	2 eggs	2	150
Meal 2	1 oz. almonds, roasted and salted	4	180
	½ cup cantaloupe, cubed	6	25
	½ cup cottage cheese, 1% fat	5	80
Meal 3	1 Free Foods Salad	FREE	FREE
	6 oz. chopped sirloin, broiled	0	323
Meal 4	1 Curves Shake or similar protein shake (see page 59)	FREE	FREE
Meal 5	1 cup broccoli, steamed	FREE	FREE
	1 tsp. butter	0	34
	8 oz. scallops, marinated in	5	200
	Seafood Marinade (see page 301)	2	30
	1 serving Vegetable Soup (see page 291)	5	85
Meal 6	2 plums, medium	18	72
	1 oz. Havarti cheese	0	120

Week 1 Wednesday

Meal		Carbs	Calories
Meal 1	¼ cup blueberries	7	27
	8 oz. yogurt, plain	18	150
Meal 2	1 Curves Shake or similar protein shake (see page 59)	FREE	FREE
Meal 3	1 serving Spinach Salad with Orange Vinaigrette (see page 288)	3	101
	8 oz. chicken breast, broiled	0	248
Meal 4	2 RyKrisp crackers	11	60
	4.25-oz. can sardines	2	190
	4 oz. V8 juice	5	23
Meal 5	1 cup zucchini, sautéed in	FREE	FREE
	1 Tbsp. olive oil	0	120
	1 serving Lemony Cauliflower (see page 304)	0	75
	1 serving Buffalo Meatballs (see page 292)	2	243
Meal 6	3 oz. ham, lean	0	120
	1 oz. Havarti cheese	0	120

Week 1 Thursday

Meal		Carbs	Calories
Meal 1	1 piece Holland rusk dry toast	6	30
	2 sausage links	0	134
	2 eggs	2	150
Meal 2	2 Keebler Harvest Bakery Multigrain Crackers	11	70
	2 Tbsp. vegetable cream cheese	2	90
Meal 3	½ cup asparagus	FREE	FREE
	½ cup mushrooms	FREE	FREE
	½ cup onion	FREE	FREE
	½ cup snow peas	FREE	FREE
	8 oz. shrimp, sautéed in	0	240
	1 Tbsp. olive oil	0	120
Meal 4	1 Curves Shake or similar protein shake (see page 59)	FREE	FREE
Meal 5	1 Free Foods Salad	FREE	FREE
	1 serving Beef Tenderloin with Blue Cheese (see page 297)	1	383
Meal 6	½ banana	13	53
	1 oz. cheddar cheese	0	110

Week 1 Friday

Meal		Carbs	Calories
Meal 1	½ cup strawberries	6	23
	4 oz. yogurt, plain	9	75
Meal 2	1 Curves Shake or similar protein shake (see page 59)	FREE	FREE
Meal 3	1 cup zucchini, sauteed in	FREE	FREE
	1 Tbsp. olive oil	0	120
	1 Free Foods Salad	FREE	FREE
	8-oz. pork chop, lean, broiled	0	300
Meal 4	3 oz. ham, lean	0	120
	1 oz. cheddar cheese	0	110
Meal 5	2 Keebler Harvest Bakery Multigrain Crackers	11	70
	1 serving Vegetable Soup (see page 291)	5	85
Meal 6	1 serving Tuna Salad (see page 295)	3	258

Week 1 Saturday

Meal		Carbs	Calories
Meal 1	1 slice bread, whole-wheat	12	70
	3 sausage links	0	200
	1 oz. Havarti cheese	0	120
Meal 2	1 Curves Shake or similar protein shake (see page 59)	FREE	FREE
Meal 3	1 serving Chicken Fajitas (see page 293)	1	280
	½ cup refried beans	25	120
Meal 4	1 oz. almonds, roasted and salted	4	180
Meal 5	1 serving Tofu Stir-Fry (see page 300)	2	340
Meal 6	1 serving Italian Soda (see page 307)	0	100

Week 1 Sunday

Meal		Carbs	Calories
Meal 1	3 sausage links	0	200
	2 eggs	2	150
Meal 2	½ cup cantaloupe, cubed	6	25
	½ cup cottage cheese, 1% fat	5	80
Meal 3	1 cup broccoli, steamed	FREE	FREE
	1 Tbsp. butter	0	102
	1 Cornish hen, roasted, no skin	0	300
	1 Free Foods Salad	FREE	FREE
Meal 4	1 serving Spicy Zucchini Boats (see page 305)	2	195
Meal 5	1 cup spinach	FREE	FREE
	8 oz. shrimp, sauteed in	0	240
	1 Tbsp. olive oil	0	120
	1 apple, small	20	80
Meal 6	1 Curves Shake or similar protein shake (see page 59)	FREE	FREE

Week 2 Monday

Meal		Carbs	Calories
Meal 1	½ cup strawberries	6	23
	½ cup cottage cheese, 1% fat	5	80
Meal 2	1 Curves Shake or similar protein shake (see page 59)	FREE	FREE
Meal 3	1 cup carrots, cooked	11	48
	1 tsp. butter	0	34
	6 oz. ground beef, 93% lean, broiled	0	240
Meal 4	1 Free Foods Salad	FREE	FREE
	1 serving Buffalo Meatballs (see page 292)	2	243
Meal 5	1 serving Chinese Vegetables (see page 303)	8	160
	8-oz. chicken breast, broiled	0	248
	4 oz. V8 juice	5	23
Meal 6	3 oz. ham, lean	0	120
	1 oz. Havarti cheese	0	120

Week 2 Tuesday		*Carbs*	*Calories*
Meal 1	3 oz. ham, lean	0	120
	2 eggs	2	150
	1 Tbsp. butter	0	102
Meal 2	1 oz. cashews, roasted and salted	7	170
	½ cup cantaloupe, cubed	6	25
	½ cup cottage cheese, 1% fat	5	80
Meal 3	1 serving Greek Salad (see page 288)	6	348
Meal 4	1 Curves Shake or similar protein shake (see page 59)	FREE	FREE
Meal 5	1 cup cauliflower, steamed	FREE	FREE
	1 Tbsp. butter	0	102
	1 serving French Onion Soup (see page 290)	3	145
	8 oz. trout, broiled	0	373
Meal 6	1 orange, medium	16	65

Week 2 Wednesday			
Meal 1	¼ cup blueberries	7	27
	4 oz. yogurt, plain	9	75
Meal 2	1 Curves Shake or similar protein shake (see page 59)	FREE	FREE
Meal 3	1 serving Spinach Salad with Orange Vinaigrette (see page 288)	3	101
	6-oz. flank steak, broiled	0	384
Meal 4	1 slice bread, whole-wheat	12	70
	½ Tbsp. butter	0	51
	1 serving Vegetable Soup (see page 291)	5	85
Meal 5	1 cup zucchini, sauteed in	FREE	FREE
	1 Tbsp. olive oil	0	120
	½ cup sauerkraut	FREE	FREE
	6 oz. smoked sausage, low-fat	12	330
Meal 6	2 oz. roast beef, deli	2	60
	1 oz. Havarti cheese	0	120

Week 2 Thursday

Meal		Carbs	Calories
Meal 1	1 piece Holland rusk dry toast	6	30
	3 sausage links	0	200
	2 eggs	2	150
Meal 2	2 Keebler Harvest Bakery Multigrain Crackers	11	70
	2 Tbsp. vegetable cream cheese	2	90
Meal 3	½ cup asparagus, steamed	FREE	FREE
	1 tsp. butter	0	34
	1 serving Sherry-Mushroom Chicken (see page 301)	3	288
Meal 4	1 Curves Shake or similar protein shake (see page 59)	FREE	FREE
Meal 5	½ cup peas, green, steamed	11	60
	1 tsp. butter	0	34
	1 Free Foods Salad	FREE	FREE
	6-oz. pork chop, lean, broiled	0	225
Meal 6	1 oz. cashews, roasted and salted	7	170
	½ cup watermelon, cubed	6	25
	1 oz. cheddar cheese	0	110

Week 2 Friday

Meal		Carbs	Calories
Meal 1	½ cup strawberries	6	23
	4 oz. yogurt, plain	9	75
Meal 2	1 Curves Shake or similar protein shake (see page 59)	FREE	FREE
Meal 3	1 serving Easy Frittata (see page 298)	4	325
	1 Free Foods Salad	FREE	FREE
Meal 4	½ cup brussels sprouts, steamed	FREE	FREE
	1 tsp. butter	0	34
	6-oz. lamb chop, broiled	0	548
Meal 5	1 oz. cheddar cheese	0	110
	2 Keebler Harvest Bakery Multigrain Crackers	11	70
Meal 6	1 serving Tuna Salad (see page 295)	3	258

Week 2 Saturday		Carbs	Calories
Meal 1	1 slice bread, whole-wheat	12	70
	3 sausage links	0	200
	1 oz. Havarti cheese	0	120
Meal 2	1 Curves Shake or similar protein shake (see page 59)	FREE	FREE
Meal 3	½ cup refried beans	25	120
	2 Tbsp. salsa	2	10
	6 oz. ground beef, 93% lean, broiled	0	240
	1 oz. cheddar cheese	0	110
Meal 4	1 oz. macadamia nuts	5	160
Meal 5	1 Free Foods Salad	FREE	FREE
Meal 6	1 serving Tofu Stir-Fry (see page 300)	2	340

Week 2 Sunday			
Meal 1	4 oz. V8 juice	5	23
	3 sausage links	0	200
	2 eggs	2	150
Meal 2	½ cup cantaloupe, cubed	6	25
	½ cup cottage cheese, 1% fat	5	80
Meal 3	1 cup green beans	8	40
	1 tsp. butter	0	34
	6-oz. chicken breast, broiled	0	186
	1 Tbsp. Parmesan cheese, grated	0	28
	1 Free Foods Salad	FREE	FREE
Meal 4	4 oz. wine, rosé	6	120
	½ banana	13	53
	2 oz. Havarti cheese	0	240
Meal 5	1 cup spinach	FREE	FREE
	8 oz. shrimp, sauteed in	0	240
	1 Tbsp. olive oil	0	120
Meal 6	1 Curves Shake or similar protein shake (see page 59)	FREE	FREE

Week 3
Monday

		Carbs	Calories
Meal 1	½ cup cottage cheese, 1% fat	5	80
	½ cup strawberries	6	23
Meal 2	1 Curves Shake or similar protein shake (see page 59)	FREE	FREE
Meal 3	1 cup carrots, cooked	11	48
	1 tsp. butter	0	34
	1 Free Foods Salad	FREE	FREE
	6 oz. ground beef, 93% lean, broiled	0	240
Meal 4	2 RyKrisp crackers	11	60
	1 serving Tuna Salad (see page 295)	3	258
Meal 5	1 cup broccoli, steamed	FREE	FREE
	1 tsp. butter	0	34
	8-oz. chicken breast, broiled	0	248
	1 Tbsp. barbeque sauce	6	25
	1 serving Creamy Coleslaw (see page 289)	3	78
Meal 6	3 oz. ham, lean	0	120
	1 oz. Havarti cheese	0	120

Week 3
Tuesday

		Carbs	Calories
Meal 1	3 oz. ham, lean	0	120
	2 eggs	2	150
	1 tsp. butter	0	34
Meal 2	½ cup cantaloupe, cubed	6	25
	½ cup cottage cheese, 1% fat	5	80
Meal 3	1 serving Greek Salad (see page 288)	6	348
Meal 4	1 Curves Shake or similar protein shake (see page 59)	FREE	FREE
Meal 5	1 cup green beans	8	40
	1 tsp. butter	0	34
	1 serving Lemony Cauliflower (see page 304)	0	75
	8 oz. orange roughy, broiled	0	216
Meal 6	1 apple, small	20	80
	1 oz. Havarti cheese	0	120

Week 3 Wednesday

Meal		Carbs	Calories
Meal 1	¼ cup blueberries	7	27
	8 oz. yogurt, plain	18	150
Meal 2	1 Curves Shake or similar protein shake (see page 59)	FREE	FREE
Meal 3	1 Free Foods Salad	FREE	FREE
	6-oz. pork chop, lean, broiled	0	225
Meal 4	1 serving Italian Soda (see page 307)	0	100
	2 oz. pistachio nuts, in shells	7	170
Meal 5	1 cup zucchini, sauteed in	FREE	FREE
	1 Tbsp. olive oil	0	120
	½ cup sauerkraut	FREE	FREE
	6 oz. smoked sausage, low-fat	12	330
Meal 6	2 oz. ham, lean	0	80
	1 oz. Havarti cheese	0	120

Week 3 Thursday

Meal		Carbs	Calories
Meal 1	1 piece Holland rusk dry toast	6	30
	3 sausage links	0	200
	2 eggs	2	150
Meal 2	2 Keebler Harvest Bakery Multigrain Crackers	11	70
	2 Tbsp. vegetable cream cheese	2	90
Meal 3	½ cup asparagus, steamed	FREE	FREE
	1 tsp. butter	0	34
	1 serving Sherry-Mushroom Chicken (see page 301)	3	288
Meal 4	1 Curves Shake or similar protein shake (see page 59)	FREE	FREE
Meal 5	1 Free Foods Salad	FREE	FREE
	1 serving Beef & Vegetable Stew (see page 296)	8	256
Meal 6	1 oz. cashews, roasted and salted	7	170
	½ cup watermelon, cubed	6	25
	1 oz. cheddar cheese	0	110

Week 3 Friday

Meal		Carbs	Calories
Meal 1	4 strips bacon	0	147
	2 eggs	2	150
Meal 2	1 Curves Shake or similar protein shake (see page 59)	FREE	FREE
Meal 3	1 Free Foods Salad	FREE	FREE
	1 serving Easy Frittata (see page 298)	4	325
Meal 4	1 slice bread, whole-wheat	12	70
	1 oz. cheddar cheese	0	110
	4 oz. roast beef, deli	4	120
	1 Tbsp. light mayonnaise	1	50
	1 serving Vegetable Soup (see page 291)	5	85
Meal 5	½ cup cantaloupe, cubed	6	25
	½ cup cottage cheese, 1% fat	5	80
Meal 6	2 Turkey-Lettuce Wraps (see page 293)	12	166

Week 3 Saturday

Meal		Carbs	Calories
Meal 1	1 slice bread, whole-wheat	12	70
	3 sausage links	0	200
	1 oz. Havarti cheese	0	120
Meal 2	1 Curves Shake or similar protein shake (see page 59)	FREE	FREE
Meal 3	1 serving Chicken Fajitas (see page 293)	1	280
	½ cup refried beans	25	120
Meal 4	1 oz. cashews, roasted and salted	7	170
Meal 5	1 serving Parmesan Vegetable Stir-Fry (see page 304)	0	175
	6 oz. halibut, broiled	0	240
Meal 6	1 Free Foods Salad	FREE	FREE

Week 3 Sunday		Carbs	Calories
Meal 1	4 oz. V8 juice	5	23
	3 sausage links	0	200
	2 eggs	2	150
Meal 2	½ cup cantaloupe, cubed	6	25
	½ cup cottage cheese, 1% fat	5	80
Meal 3	½ cup snow peas, steamed	FREE	FREE
	1 tsp. butter	0	34
	6 oz. chicken breast, broiled	0	186
	1 orange, medium	16	65
Meal 4	4 oz. wine, rosé	6	120
	1 oz. Havarti cheese	0	120
Meal 5	1 cup spinach	FREE	FREE
	1 cup mushrooms	FREE	FREE
	8 oz. scallops sauteed in	5	200
	1 Tbsp. olive oil	0	120
	1 Free Foods Salad	FREE	FREE
Meal 6	1 Curves Shake or similar protein shake (see page 59)	FREE	FREE

Week 4 Monday			
Meal 1	½ cup strawberries	6	23
	½ cup cottage cheese, 1% fat	5	80
Meal 2	1 Curves Shake or similar protein shake (see page 59)	FREE	FREE
Meal 3	1 cup carrots, cooked	11	48
	1 tsp. butter	0	34
	6 oz. ground beef, 93% lean, broiled	0	240
	1 plum, medium	9	36
Meal 4	1 serving French Onion Soup (see page 290)	3	145
	1 Tbsp. Parmesan cheese, grated	0	28
	1 serving Italian Soda (see page 307)	0	100
Meal 5	1 cup cauliflower, steamed	FREE	FREE
	1 tsp. butter	0	34
	1 Free Foods Salad	FREE	FREE
	1 serving Spicy Chili Pork Chops (see page 302)	4	219
Meal 6	4 oz. wine, rosé	6	120
	3 oz. ham, lean	0	120
	1 oz. Monterey Jack cheese	0	110

Week 4 Tuesday

Meal		Carbs	Calories
Meal 1	3 oz. ham, lean	0	120
	2 eggs	2	150
	1 tsp. butter	0	34
Meal 2	½ cup cantaloupe, cubed	6	25
	½ cup cottage cheese, 1% fat	5	80
Meal 3	1 serving Greek Salad (see page 288)	6	348
	1 serving Frozen Chocolate Mousse (see page 306)	9	127
Meal 4	1 Curves Shake or similar protein shake (see page 59)	FREE	FREE
Meal 5	¼ cup corn, whole-kernel	7	3
	1 cup zucchini, sauteed in	FREE	FREE
	1 Tbsp. olive oil	0	120
	1 serving Jamaican Seafood Medley (see page 299)	6	283
Meal 6	2 Keebler Harvest Bakery Multigrain Crackers	11	70
	2 oz. cheddar cheese	0	220

Week 4 Wednesday

Meal		Carbs	Calories
Meal 1	¼ cup blueberries	7	27
	4 oz. yogurt, plain	9	75
Meal 2	1 Curves Shake or similar protein shake (see page 59)	FREE	FREE
Meal 3	½ cup red bell pepper	FREE	FREE
	½ cup zucchini, sauteed in	FREE	FREE
	1 Tbsp. olive oil	0	120
	½ cup sauerkraut	FREE	FREE
	6-oz. pork chop, lean, broiled	0	225
Meal 4	1 serving Italian Stuffed Mushrooms (see page 294)	13	177
	8 oz. V8 juice	10	46
Meal 5	1 Free Foods Salad	FREE	FREE
	1 serving Beef Tenderloin with Blue Cheese (see page 297)	1	383
Meal 6	3 oz. ham, lean	0	120
	1 oz. Monterey Jack cheese	0	110

Week 4 Thursday		Carbs	Calories
Meal 1	1 piece Holland rusk dry toast	6	30
	3 sausage links	0	200
	2 eggs	2	150
Meal 2	2 Keebler Harvest Bakery Multigrain Crackers	11	70
	2 Tbsp. vegetable cream cheese	2	90
	1 cup watermelon, cubed	12	50
Meal 3	1 cup broccoli, steamed	FREE	FREE
	1 tsp. butter	0	34
	1 Tbsp. blue cheese	0	48
	6-oz. chicken breast, broiled	0	186
Meal 4	1 Curves Shake or similar protein shake (see page 59)	FREE	FREE
Meal 5	1 Free Foods Salad	FREE	FREE
	1 serving Beef & Vegetable Stew (see page 296)	8	256
Meal 6	1 oz. peanuts, dry-roasted	5	160
	1 oz. cheddar cheese	0	110

Week 4 Friday			
Meal 1	3 oz. ham, lean	0	120
	2 eggs	2	150
	1 tsp. butter	0	34
Meal 2	1 Curves Shake or similar protein shake (see page 59)	FREE	FREE
Meal 3	2 Turkey-Lettuce Wraps (see page 293)	12	166
	1/2 cup strawberries	6	23
Meal 4	2 RyKrisp crackers	11	60
	2 oz. cheddar cheese	0	220
Meal 5	1 cup asparagus	FREE	FREE
	1 tsp. butter	0	34
	1 Free Foods Salad	FREE	FREE
	8-oz. tuna steak (fresh), marinated in	0	246
	Seafood Marinade (see page 301)	2	30
Meal 6	1/2 cup cantaloupe, cubed	6	25
	1/2 cup cottage cheese, 1% fat	5	80

Week 4 Saturday

Meal		Carbs	Calories
Meal 1	1 slice bread, whole-wheat	12	70
	3 sausage links	0	200
	1 oz. Monterey Jack cheese	0	110
Meal 2	1 Curves Shake or similar protein shake (see page 59)	FREE	FREE
Meal 3	½ cup refried beans	25	120
	2 Tbsp. salsa	2	10
	6 oz. ground beef, 93% lean, broiled	0	240
	1 oz. cheddar cheese	0	110
Meal 4	1 serving Spicy Zucchini Boats (see page 305)	2	195
	6 oz. salmon, broiled	0	310
Meal 5	1 Free Foods Salad	FREE	FREE
Meal 6	1 oz. peanuts, dry-roasted	5	160

Week 4 Sunday

Meal		Carbs	Calories
Meal 1	4 strips bacon	0	147
	2 eggs	2	150
Meal 2	½ cup cantaloupe, cubed	6	25
	½ cup cottage cheese, 1% fat	5	80
Meal 3	½ cup snow peas, steamed	FREE	FREE
	1 tsp. butter	0	34
	6-oz. chicken breast, broiled	0	186
	1 orange, medium	16	65
Meal 4	2 RyKrisp crackers	11	60
	2 oz. Monterey Jack cheese	0	220
	4 oz. wine, rosé	6	120
Meal 5	1 cup mushrooms	FREE	FREE
	1 cup spinach	FREE	FREE
	8 oz. orange roughy, sautéed in	0	216
	1 Tbsp. olive oil	0	120
	1 Free Foods Salad	FREE	FREE
Meal 6	1 Curves Shake or similar protein shake (see page 59)	FREE	FREE

Week 5 Monday		Carbs	Calories
Meal 1	1 slice bread, whole-wheat	12	70
	2 oz. turkey breast, deli	2	60
	1 oz. Swiss cheese	0	110
	1 Tbsp. light mayonnaise	1	50
Meal 2	½ cup baby carrots	5	24
	½ cup cottage cheese, 1% fat	5	80
Meal 3	1 serving French Onion Soup (see page 290)	3	145
	6 oz. ground beef, 93% lean, broiled	0	240
Meal 4	1 oz. macadamia nuts	5	160
	½ cup grapes, seedless	14	57
Meal 5	1 cup broccoli, steamed	FREE	FREE
	1 tsp. butter	0	34
	1 Free Foods Salad	FREE	FREE
	1 serving Spicy Chili Pork Chops (see page 302)	4	219
Meal 6	1 Curves Shake or similar protein shake (see page 59)	FREE	FREE

Week 5 Tuesday			
Meal 1	3 oz. ham, lean	0	120
	2 eggs	2	150
Meal 2	½ cup strawberries	6	23
	½ cup cottage cheese, 1% fat	5	80
Meal 3	1 slice bread, whole-wheat	12	70
	½ Tbsp. butter	0	51
	6-oz. chicken breast, broiled	0	186
	1 serving Spinach Salad with Orange Vinaigrette (see page 288)	3	101
Meal 4	1 Curves Shake or similar protein shake (see page 59)	FREE	FREE
Meal 5	1 cup zucchini, sauteed in	FREE	FREE
	1 Tbsp. olive oil	0	120
	1 serving Jamaican Seafood Medley (see page 299)	6	283
	1 serving Frozen Chocolate Mousse (see page 306)	9	127
Meal 6	1 oz. almonds, roasted and salted	4	180
	1 oz. cheddar cheese	0	110

Week 5 Wednesday

Meal	Food	Carbs	Calories
Meal 1	4 oz. yogurt, plain	9	75
Meal 2	1 Curves Shake or similar protein shake (see page 59)	FREE	FREE
Meal 3	½ cup refried beans	25	120
	2 Tbsp. salsa	2	10
	6 oz. ground beef, 93% lean, broiled	0	240
	1 oz. cheddar cheese	0	110
Meal 4	1 serving Spicy Zucchini Boats (see page 305)	2	195
	1 serving Vegetable Soup (see page 291)	5	85
Meal 5	1 Free Foods Salad	FREE	FREE
	8-oz. pork chop, lean, broiled	0	300
Meal 6	2 oz. roast beef, deli	2	60
	1 oz. Swiss cheese	0	110

Week 5 Thursday

Meal	Food	Carbs	Calories
Meal 1	4 strips bacon	0	147
	2 eggs	2	150
Meal 2	2 Keebler Harvest Bakery Multigrain Crackers	11	70
	2 Tbsp. vegetable cream cheese	2	90
	1 cup watermelon, cubed	12	50
Meal 3	½ cup peas, green, steamed	11	60
	1 tsp. butter	0	34
	1 Tbsp. blue cheese	0	48
	6-oz. chicken breast, broiled	0	186
Meal 4	1 Curves Shake or similar protein shake (see page 59)	FREE	FREE
Meal 5	1 Free Foods Salad	FREE	FREE
	6 oz. sirloin steak, broiled	0	323
Meal 6	4 oz. wine, rosé	6	120
	1 oz. cheddar cheese	0	110

Week 5 Friday		Carbs	Calories
Meal 1	1 piece Holland rusk dry toast	6	30
	3 sausage links	0	200
	1 egg	1	75
Meal 2	1 Curves Shake or similar protein shake (see page 59)	FREE	FREE
Meal 3	1 serving Creamy Coleslaw (see page 289)	3	78
	6 oz. ground beef, 93% lean, broiled	0	240
	1 Tbsp. barbeque sauce	6	25
Meal 4	1 serving Italian Stuffed Mushrooms (see page 294)	13	177
Meal 5	1 Free Foods Salad	FREE	FREE
	1 serving Lemony Cauliflower (see page 304)	0	75
	8 oz. shrimp, sauteed in	0	240
	1 Tbsp. olive oil	0	120
Meal 6	½ cup strawberries	6	23
	½ cup cottage cheese, 1% fat	5	80

Week 5 Saturday			
Meal 1	1 slice bread, whole-wheat	12	70
	3 sausage links	0	200
	1 oz. cheddar cheese	0	110
Meal 2	1 Curves Shake or similar protein shake (see page 59)	FREE	FREE
Meal 3	1 Free Foods Salad	FREE	FREE
Meal 4	½ cup snow peas, steamed	FREE	FREE
	1 tsp. butter	0	34
	6-oz. chicken breast, broiled	0	186
Meal 5	1 serving Chinese Vegetables (see page 303)	8	160
	8 oz. red snapper, broiled	0	226
Meal 6	½ cup French vanilla ice cream	15	160
	1 oz. peanuts, dry-roasted	5	160
	½ cup strawberries	6	23

Week 5
Sunday

		Carbs	Calories
Meal 1	4 strips bacon	0	147
	2 eggs	2	150
Meal 2	½ cup watermelon, cubed	6	25
	½ cup cottage cheese, 1% fat	5	80
Meal 3	1 cup green beans	8	40
	1 tsp. butter	0	34
	½ cup sauerkraut	FREE	FREE
	8 oz. smoked sausage, low-fat	16	440
Meal 4	2 Keebler Harvest Bakery Multigrain Crackers	11	70
	2 oz. Swiss cheese	0	220
Meal 5	1 Free Foods Salad	FREE	FREE
	1 serving Sherry-Mushroom Chicken (see page 301)	3	288
Meal 6	1 Curves Shake or similar protein shake (see page 59)	FREE	FREE

Curves Profile

TANYA G.

MINOT, NORTH DAKOTA

Since I joined Curves in September 1999, I went from a size 26 to a size 8 and lost 130 pounds. I've dieted and lost weight before, but with Curves it was the first time I'd ever toned up my body, and it's the first time I've kept the weight off. I had never really exercised before, other than taking a walk with my family, which really isn't exercise. When I first walked into Curves, I panicked and thought, *This is neat but, man, it looks like a lot of work. I'll never last!* After I started at Curves, I saw that it was really pretty easy, the pounds were rolling off me, and I felt great. That was all the motivation I needed to keep going. Now I can't imagine my life without Curves.

Since I've lost all the weight, my life has changed a great deal. You wouldn't think that being overweight would make such a difference, but it does. I'm a hairdresser, and I always talked a lot and had lots of friends, but now my clients treat me differently. At first, I thought, *Why didn't she like me before? I was the same person.* Now I realize that I wasn't the same person, because when you're heavier you're not as outgoing or sure of yourself.

I have a lot more energy than I used to have. I no longer have to stop and catch my breath after doing a simple activity. I used to go to bed at eight or nine at night because I was exhausted, but after a few weeks at Curves, I would be able to stay up so late that my husband would ask, "Are you *ever* coming to bed?" I just had so much energy, and, as a working mother, I had so many things to do that I figured I might as well do them.

I work full-time. A lot of women use that as an excuse not to exercise. I take my children to day care early so that I can have my time at Curves. I'm there from seven-thirty to eight every morning. That is the only time I consider *my* time. And it's what I enjoy doing.

I think no matter what you do as far as exercise, you still have to watch what you eat. And so many people think that because you go and work out you can eat whatever you want all the time. You can't. So eating healthy food along with exercising is definitely the way to go. I eat whatever I want—I don't deny myself anything—but I am more aware of portion control, and I don't feel like I have to clean my plate at every meal.

I have two children, and I'm able to do a lot more things with them now. When I was heavy, I would take my oldest daughter to the park and just sit on the bench and watch her play. I couldn't do much more. Now I'm out there playing right along with my children. I am very grateful to Curves for that.

What's really great is that now I can go and buy the clothes that I really like, and I don't have to look for clothes that hide my body or make me look thinner. I even went into the junior department recently and bought some leather pants because they were cool and I thought it would be hip for a hairdresser to wear them.

It took me a long time to get used to my new body. I used to catch my reflection in the mirror and wonder, *Who is that slim woman?* It took me the longest time to realize that the woman in the mirror was me!

CHAPTER 6

THE CALORIE-
SENSITIVE PLAN

n the pages that follow, you will find seven weeks of sample menus for the Calorie-Sensitive Plan: two weeks of Phase 1 menus and five weeks of Phase 2 menus. You can follow these menus, or you can change the order of the meals as you see fit. You may find that you like some meals but dislike others. Use the blank menu forms in your Daily Meal Planner (see page 311) to customize the meal plan to reflect your tastes. As long as you stay within your calorie and carbohydrate guidelines, you can be as creative as you like.

In the Daily Meal Planner, you will also find weekly shopping lists for these menus and recipes for the special Curves meals listed in the menus. Please note that the ingredients for the special recipes are not included in the weekly shopping lists, for the simple reason that not everyone likes to cook. If you choose to make these dishes, you must add the ingredients to your weekly shopping list.

Before you get started, let me review the basic requirements for each phase.

Phase 1

- If you have less than 20 pounds to lose, follow Phase 1 for only 1 week.
- If you have more than 20 pounds to lose, stay on Phase 1 for two weeks.
- At the end of Phase 1, move on to Phase 2.

You can eat *1,200 calories* daily and no more than *60 grams of carbohydrates.* Try to consume about 40 percent of your daily calories from protein. Be sure to stick to the correct protein portion sizes or you'll risk eating too many calories. You are also allowed to eat unlimited amounts of Free Foods and your one protein shake daily.

PROBLEM: What If You Don't Lose Enough?
Although most women will lose a substantial amount of weight on Phase 1 (between six and 10 pounds), a small minority may not.

- If you have not lost at least three pounds in the first week, or have lost fewer than two pounds in the second week, your metabolism is stuck in low gear. You need to turn it up before you can lose weight. The solution? The Metabolic Tune-Up (see page 35), where you will eat more food to get your metabolism moving again.

Phase 2

Stay on Phase 2 until you reach your desired weight, you plateau, or you want a break from dieting.

Increase your total caloric intake to 1,600, mainly in the form of protein. That means bigger servings of meat, chicken, and fish. Continue to eat 60 grams of carbohydrate daily, along with unlimited quantities of Free Foods and your one protein shake daily.

Expect to lose about two pounds of body fat each week for the first few weeks and one pound every week thereafter. As long as you are steadily losing weight, stay on Phase 2 until you reach your desired weight.

PROBLEM: What If You Plateau?

If, after a few weeks or even months on Phase 2, you stop losing one pound a week before you reach your goal, you need to change what you are doing.

- If you have stopped losing weight, it's a sign that you need a Metabolic Tune-Up (see page 35). After you have raised your metabolism, go back to Phase 1 and cycle through the program again.
- People who want to lose 50 or more pounds may have to cycle through the phases several times before they can achieve their desired goal, periodically stopping for a Metabolic Tune-Up (see page 35).

PROBLEM: What If You Want Time Off?

If you need some time off from your weight-loss plan, give yourself a Metabolic Tune-Up (see page 35). When you are ready to resume your weight-loss regimen, go back to Phase 1.

KEEPING TRACK · Count your calories and carbohydrates for each meal, and record the total on your Daily Meal Planner (see page 311).

Phase 1 Week 1 Monday

		Carbs	Calories
Meal 1	½ cup cottage cheese, 1% fat	5	80
	½ cup strawberries	6	23
Meal 2	1 Curves Shake or similar protein shake (see page 59)	FREE	FREE
Meal 3	1 Free Foods Salad	FREE	FREE
	4 oz. ground beef, 93% lean, broiled	0	160
Meal 4	2 RyKrisp crackers	11	60
	2 Tbsp. vegetable cream cheese	2	90
Meal 5	4-oz. chicken breast, broiled	0	124
	1 serving Parmesan Vegetable Stir-Fry (see page 304)	0	175
Meal 6	1 apple, small	20	80
	3 oz. ham, lean	0	120

Week 1 Tuesday

		Carbs	Calories
Meal 1	1 slice bread, whole-wheat	12	70
	1 egg	1	75
	1 tomato, sliced	5.7	26
Meal 2	½ cup cantaloupe, cubed	6	25
	½ cup cottage cheese, 1% fat	5	80
Meal 3	1 Free Foods Salad	FREE	FREE
	4 oz. turkey breast, deli	4	120
Meal 4	1 Curves Shake or similar protein shake (see page 59)	FREE	FREE
Meal 5	½ cup broccoli, steamed	FREE	FREE
	½ cup cauliflower, steamed	FREE	FREE
	1 Tbsp. butter	0	102
	4-oz. sirloin steak, broiled	0	215
Meal 6	1 oz. Havarti cheese	0	120
	1 oz. peanuts, dry-roasted	5	160

Week 1 Wednesday		Carbs	Calories
Meal 1	¼ cup blueberries	7	27
	4 oz. yogurt, plain	9	75
Meal 2	1 Curves Shake or similar protein shake (see page 59)	FREE	FREE
Meal 3	1 Free Foods Salad	FREE	FREE
	4 oz. roast beef, deli	4	120
Meal 4	2 RyKrisp crackers	11	60
	1 serving Tuna Salad (see page 295)	3	258
Meal 5	4-oz. pork chop, lean, broiled	0	150
	½ cup zucchini, sauteed in	FREE	FREE
	½ Tbsp. olive oil	0	60
Meal 6	1 oz. cheddar cheese	0	110
	1 medium dill pickle	FREE	FREE
	3 oz. ham, lean	0	120

Week 1 Thursday			
Meal 1	1 slice bread, whole-wheat	12	70
	1 egg	1	75
	2 sausage links	0	134
Meal 2	½ cup baby carrots	5	24
	½ cup cottage cheese, 1% fat	5	80
Meal 3	1 Free Foods Salad	FREE	FREE
	2.8 oz. (one small can) tuna, packed in water	0	100
Meal 4	1 Curves Shake or similar protein shake (see page 59)	FREE	FREE
Meal 5	1 serving Chicken Fajitas (see page 293)	1	280
Meal 6	1 oz. Havarti cheese	0	120
	1 orange, medium	16	65

Week 1 Friday

Meal		Carbs	Calories
Meal 1	1 slice bread, whole-wheat	12	70
	½ grapefruit	12	46
	3 oz. ham, lean	0	120
Meal 2	½ cup cantaloupe, cubed	6	25
	½ cup cottage cheese, 1% fat	5	80
Meal 3	½ cup brussels sprouts, steamed	FREE	FREE
	1 tsp. butter	0	34
	4 oz. salmon, broiled	0	207
Meal 4	1 Curves Shake or similar protein shake (see page 59)	FREE	FREE
Meal 5	1 Free Foods Salad	FREE	FREE
Meal 6	2 celery stalks	FREE	FREE
	1 oz. cheddar cheese	0	110
	1 oz. peanuts, dry-roasted	5	160

Week 1 Saturday

Meal		Carbs	Calories
Meal 1	1 slice bread, whole-wheat	12	70
	½ Tbsp. butter	0	51
	2 sausage links	0	200
Meal 2	1 Curves Shake or similar protein shake (see page 59)	FREE	FREE
Meal 3	1 Free Foods Salad	FREE	FREE
Meal 4	1 medium dill pickle	FREE	FREE
	4 oz. ground beef, 93% lean, broiled	0	160
	8 oz. V8 juice	10	46
Meal 5	8 oz. cod fillet, broiled	0	186
	1 serving French Onion Soup (see page 290)	3	145
	½ cup peas, green, steamed	11	60
Meal 6	2 Tbsp. blueberries	4	14
	4 oz. yogurt, plain	9	75

Week 1 Sunday		Carbs	Calories
Meal 1	½ grapefruit	12	46
	3 sausage links	0	200
Meal 2	4-oz. chicken breast, broiled	0	124
	1 serving Vegetable Soup (see page 291)	5	85
Meal 3	1 Free Foods Salad	FREE	FREE
Meal 4	½ cup cantaloupe, cubed	6	25
	½ cup cottage cheese, 1% fat	5	80
	2 Keebler Harvest Bakery Multigrain Crackers	11	70
Meal 5	½ cup cauliflower, steamed	FREE	FREE
	8 oz. orange roughy, sauteed in	0	216
	1 Tbsp. olive oil	0	120
	1 cup spinach	FREE	FREE
Meal 6	1 Curves Shake or similar protein shake (see page 59)	FREE	FREE

Week 2 Monday			
Meal 1	½ cup cottage cheese, 1% fat	5	80
	½ cup strawberries	6	23
Meal 2	1 Curves Shake or similar protein shake (see page 59)	FREE	FREE
Meal 3	1 Free Foods Salad	FREE	FREE
	4 oz. ground beef, 93% lean, broiled	0	160
Meal 4	2 RyKrisp crackers	11	60
	2 Tbsp. vegetable cream cheese	2	90
Meal 5	4 oz. chicken breast, broiled	0	124
	1 serving Parmesan Vegetable Stir-Fry (see page 304)	0	175
Meal 6	1 apple, small	20	80
	3 oz. ham, lean	0	120

Week 2 Tuesday

Meal		Carbs	Calories
Meal 1	1 slice bread, whole-wheat	12	70
	1 egg	1	75
	1 tomato, sliced	5.7	26
Meal 2	½ cup cantaloupe, cubed	6	25
	½ cup cottage cheese, 1% fat	5	80
Meal 3	1 Free Foods Salad	FREE	FREE
	4 oz. turkey breast, deli	4	120
Meal 4	1 Curves Shake or similar protein shake (see page 59)	FREE	FREE
Meal 5	½ cup broccoli, steamed	FREE	FREE
	½ cup cauliflower, steamed	FREE	FREE
	1 Tbsp. butter	0	102
	4 oz. sirloin steak, broiled	0	215
Meal 6	1 oz. Havarti cheese	0	120
	1 oz. peanuts, dry-roasted	5	160

Week 2 Wednesday

Meal		Carbs	Calories
Meal 1	¼ cup blueberries	7	27
	4 oz. yogurt, plain	9	75
Meal 2	1 Curves Shake or similar protein shake (see page 59)	FREE	FREE
Meal 3	1 Free Foods Salad	FREE	FREE
	4 oz. roast beef, deli	4	120
Meal 4	2 RyKrisp crackers	11	60
	1 serving Tuna Salad (see page 295)	3	258
Meal 5	4-oz. pork chop, lean, broiled	0	150
	½ cup zucchini, sauteed in	FREE	FREE
	½ Tbsp. olive oil	0	60
Meal 6	1 oz. cheddar cheese	0	110
	1 medium dill pickle	FREE	FREE
	3 oz. ham, lean	0	120

Week 2 Thursday		Carbs	Calories
Meal 1	1 slice bread, whole-wheat	12	70
	1 egg	1	75
	2 sausage links	0	134
Meal 2	½ cup baby carrots	4	24
	½ cup cottage cheese, 1% fat	5	80
Meal 3	1 Free Foods Salad	FREE	FREE
	2.8 oz. (one small can) tuna, packed in water	0	100
Meal 4	1 Curves Shake or similar protein shake (see page 59)	FREE	FREE
Meal 5	1 serving Chicken Fajitas (see page 293)	1	280
Meal 6	1 oz. Havarti cheese	0	120
	1 orange, medium	16	65

Week 2 Friday			
Meal 1	1 slice bread, whole-wheat	12	70
	½ grapefruit	12	46
	3 oz. ham, lean	0	120
Meal 2	½ cup cantaloupe, cubed	6	25
	½ cottage cheese, 1% fat	5	80
Meal 3	½ cup brussels sprouts, steamed	FREE	FREE
	1 tsp. butter	0	34
	4 oz. salmon, broiled	0	207
Meal 4	1 Curves Shake or similar protein shake (see page 59)	FREE	FREE
Meal 5	1 Free Foods Salad	FREE	FREE
Meal 6	2 celery stalks	FREE	FREE
	1 oz. cheddar cheese	0	110
	1 oz. peanuts, dry-roasted	5	160

Week 2 Saturday

Meal		Carbs	Calories
Meal 1	1 slice bread, whole-wheat	12	70
	½ Tbsp. butter	0	51
	3 sausage links	0	200
Meal 2	1 Curves Shake or similar protein shake (see page 59)	FREE	FREE
Meal 3	1 Free Foods Salad	FREE	FREE
Meal 4	1 medium dill pickle	FREE	FREE
	4 oz. ground beef, 93% lean, broiled	0	160
	8 oz. V8 juice	10	46
Meal 5	8 oz. cod fillet, broiled	0	186
	1 serving French Onion Soup (see page 290)	3	145
	½ cup peas, green, steamed	11	60
Meal 6	2 Tbsp. blueberries	4	14
	4 oz. yogurt, plain	9	75

Week 2 Sunday

Meal		Carbs	Calories
Meal 1	½ grapefruit	12	46
	3 sausage links	0	200
Meal 2	4-oz. chicken breast, broiled	0	124
	1 serving Vegetable Soup (see page 291)	5	85
Meal 3	1 Free Foods Salad	FREE	FREE
Meal 4	½ cup cantaloupe, cubed	6	25
	½ cup cottage cheese, 1% fat	5	80
	2 Keebler Harvest Bakery Multigrain Crackers	11	70
Meal 5	½ cup cauliflower, steamed	FREE	FREE
	8 oz. orange roughy, sauteed in	0	216
	1 Tbsp. olive oil	0	120
	1 cup spinach	FREE	FREE
Meal 6	1 Curves Shake or similar protein shake (see page 59)	FREE	FREE

Phase 2 Week 1 Monday		Carbs	Calories
Meal 1	½ cup cottage cheese, 1% fat	5	80
	½ cup strawberries	6	23
Meal 2	1 Curves Shake or similar protein shake (see page 59)	FREE	FREE
Meal 3	1 Free Foods Salad	FREE	FREE
	1 serving French Onion Soup (see page 290)	3	145
	4 oz. ground beef, 93% lean, broiled	0	160
Meal 4	2 RyKrisp crackers	11	60
	1 serving Tuna Salad (see page 295)	3	258
Meal 5	6-oz. chicken breast, broiled	0	186
	1 serving Chinese Vegetables (see page 303)	8	160
	4 oz. V8 juice	5	23
Meal 6	2 oz. ham, lean	0	80
	1 oz. Havarti cheese	0	120
	1 peach, medium	9	37

Week 1 Tuesday			
Meal 1	2 eggs	2	150
	1 tomato, sliced	5.7	26
Meal 2	1 oz. almonds, roasted and salted	4	180
	½ cup cantaloupe, cubed	6	25
	½ cup cottage cheese, 1% fat	5	80
Meal 3	6 oz. chopped sirloin, broiled	0	322
	1 Free Foods Salad	FREE	FREE
Meal 4	1 Curves Shake or similar protein shake (see page 59)	FREE	FREE
Meal 5	1 cup broccoli, steamed	FREE	FREE
	1 tsp. butter	0	34
	8 oz. scallops, marinated in	5	200
	Seafood Marinade (see page 301)	2	30
Meal 6	1 apple, small	20	80
	1 oz. Havarti cheese	0	120

Week 1 Wednesday

		Carbs	Calories
Meal 1	¼ cup blueberries	7	27
	8 oz. yogurt, plain	18	150
Meal 2	1 Curves Shake or similar protein shake (see page 59)	FREE	FREE
Meal 3	8 oz. chicken breast, broiled	0	248
	1 serving Spinach Salad with Orange Vinaigrette (see page 288)	3	101
Meal 4	2 RyKrisp crackers	11	60
	4.25-oz. can sardines	2	190
	8 oz. V8 juice	10	46
Meal 5	1 serving Buffalo Meatballs (see page 292)	2	243
	1 serving Lemony Cauliflower (see page 304)	0	75
	1 cup zucchini, sauteed in	FREE	FREE
	1 Tbsp. olive oil	0	120
Meal 6	3 oz. ham, lean	0	120
	1 oz. Havarti cheese	0	120

Week 1 Thursday

Meal 1	1 slice bread, whole-wheat	12	70
	2 eggs	2	150
	2 sausage links	0	134
Meal 2	2 Keebler Harvest Bakery Multigrain Crackers	11	70
	2 Tbsp. vegetable cream cheese	2	90
Meal 3	3 artichoke heart pieces	3	18
	½ cup asparagus	FREE	FREE
	½ cup mushrooms	FREE	FREE
	½ cup onion	FREE	FREE
	8 oz. shrimp, sauteed in	0	240
	1 Tbsp. olive oil	0	120
Meal 4	1 Curves Shake or similar protein shake (see page 59)	FREE	FREE
Meal 5	1 serving Beef Tenderloin with Blue Cheese (see page 297)	1	383
	1 Free Foods Salad	FREE	FREE
Meal 6	½ banana	13	53

		Carbs	*Calories*
Meal 1	½ cup strawberries	6	23
	8 oz. yogurt, plain	18	150
Meal 2	1 Curves Shake or similar protein shake (see page 59)	FREE	FREE
Meal 3	1 Free Foods Salad	FREE	FREE
	8-oz. pork chop, lean, broiled	0	300
	1 cup zucchini, sauteed in	FREE	FREE
	1 Tbsp. olive oil	0	120
Meal 4	1 oz. cheddar cheese	0	110
	3 oz. ham, lean	0	120
Meal 5	2 Keebler Harvest Bakery Multigrain Crackers	11	70
	2 Tbsp. vegetable cream cheese	2	90
Meal 6	1 serving Tuna Salad (see page 295)	3	258
	1 serving Vegetable Soup (see page 291)	5	85

Meal 1	1 slice bread, whole-wheat	12	70
	1 oz. Havarti cheese	0	120
	3 sausage links	0	200
Meal 2	1 Curves Shake or similar protein shake (see page 59)	FREE	FREE
Meal 3	1 serving Chicken Fajitas (see page 293)	1	280
	½ cup refried beans	25	120
Meal 4	1 oz. almonds, roasted and salted	4	180
	1 serving Italian Soda (see page 307)	0	100
Meal 5	1 serving Tofu Stir-Fry (see page 300)	2	340
Meal 6	4 oz. yogurt, plain	9	75

Week 1 Sunday

		Carbs	Calories
Meal 1	1 egg	1	75
	2 sausage links	0	134
	8 oz. V8 juice	10	46
Meal 2	½ cup cantaloupe, cubed	6	25
	½ cup cottage cheese, 1% fat	5	80
Meal 3	1 cup broccoli, steamed	FREE	FREE
	1 Tbsp. butter	0	102
	1 Cornish hen, roasted, no skin	0	300
	1 Free Foods Salad	FREE	FREE
Meal 4	2 servings Spicy Zucchini Boats (see page 305)	4	390
Meal 5	1 orange, medium	16	65
	8 oz. shrimp, sauteed in	0	240
	1 Tbsp. olive oil	0	120
	1 cup spinach	FREE	FREE
Meal 6	1 Curves Shake or similar protein shake (see page 59)	FREE	FREE

Week 2 Monday

		Carbs	Calories
Meal 1	½ cup cottage cheese, 1% fat	5	80
	½ cup strawberries	6	23
Meal 2	1 Curves Shake or similar protein shake (see page 59)	FREE	FREE
Meal 3	1 cup carrots, cooked	11	48
	1 tsp. butter	0	34
	4 oz. ground beef, 93% lean, broiled	0	160
Meal 4	1 serving Buffalo Meatballs (see page 292)	2	243
	1 Free Foods Salad	FREE	FREE
Meal 5	8-oz. chicken breast, broiled	0	248
	1 serving Chinese Vegetables (see page 303)	8	160
	8 oz. V8 juice	10	46
Meal 6	3 oz. ham, lean	0	120
	1 oz. Havarti cheese	0	120

Week 2 Tuesday		Carbs	Calories
Meal 1	2 eggs	2	150
	3 oz. ham, lean	0	120
	1 piece Holland rusk dry toast	6	30
Meal 2	½ cup cantaloupe, cubed	6	25
	1 oz. cashews, roasted and salted	7	170
	½ cup cottage cheese, 1% fat	5	80
Meal 3	1 serving Greek Salad (see page 288)	6	348
Meal 4	1 Curves Shake or similar protein shake (see page 59)	FREE	FREE
Meal 5	1 cup cauliflower, steamed	FREE	FREE
	1 Tbsp. butter	0	102
	1 serving French Onion Soup (see page 290)	3	145
	6 oz. trout, broiled	0	280
Meal 6	1 apple, small	20	80

Week 2 Wednesday			
Meal 1	¼ cup blueberries	7	27
	4 oz. yogurt, plain	9	75
Meal 2	1 Curves Shake or similar protein shake (see page 59)	FREE	FREE
Meal 3	6-oz. flank steak, broiled	0	384
	1 serving Spinach Salad with Orange Vinaigrette (see page 288)	3	101
Meal 4	1 slice bread, whole-wheat	12	70
	½ Tbsp. butter	0	51
	1 serving Vegetable Soup (see page 291)	5	85
Meal 5	½ cup sauerkraut	FREE	FREE
	6 oz. smoked sausage, low-fat	12	330
	1 cup zucchini, sauteed in	FREE	FREE
	1 Tbsp. olive oil	0	120
Meal 6	1 oz. Havarti cheese	0	120
	2 oz. roast beef, deli	2	60
	8 oz. V8 juice	10	46

Week 2 Thursday		Carbs	Calories
Meal 1	2 eggs	2	150
	1 piece Holland rusk dry toast	6	30
	3 sausage links	0	200
Meal 2	2 Keebler Harvest Bakery Multigrain Crackers	11	70
	2 Tbsp. vegetable cream cheese	2	90
Meal 3	½ cup asparagus, steamed	FREE	FREE
	1 tsp. butter	0	34
	1 serving Sherry-Mushroom Chicken (see page 301)	3	288
Meal 4	1 Curves Shake or similar protein shake (see page 59)	FREE	FREE
Meal 5	1 Free Foods Salad	FREE	FREE
	½ cup peas, green, steamed	11	60
	1 tsp. butter	0	34
	4-oz. pork chop, lean, broiled	0	150
Meal 6	1 oz. cashews, roasted and salted	7	170
	1 oz. cheddar cheese	0	110
	½ cup watermelon, cubed	6	25

Week 2 Friday			
Meal 1	½ cup strawberries	6	23
	4 oz. yogurt, plain	9	75
Meal 2	1 Curves Shake or similar protein shake (see page 59)	FREE	FREE
Meal 3	1 serving Easy Frittata (see page 298)	4	325
	1 Free Foods Salad	FREE	FREE
Meal 4	½ cup brussels sprouts, steamed	FREE	FREE
	1 tsp. butter	0	34
	4-oz. lamb chop, broiled	0	364
	1 orange, medium	16	65
Meal 5	1 oz. cheddar cheese	0	110
	2 Keebler Harvest Bakery Multigrain Crackers	11	70
Meal 6	1 serving Tuna Salad (see page 295)	3	258

Week 2 Saturday		Carbs	Calories
Meal 1	4 strips bacon	0	147
	1 slice bread, whole-wheat	12	70
	1 Tbsp. light mayonnaise	1	50
	½ tomato, sliced	3	13
Meal 2	1 Curves Shake or similar protein shake (see page 59)	FREE	FREE
Meal 3	1 oz. cheddar cheese	0	110
	6 oz. ground beef, 93% lean, broiled	0	240
	½ cup refried beans	25	120
	2 Tbsp. salsa	2	10
Meal 4	1 oz. macadamia nuts	5	160
Meal 5	1 Free Foods Salad	FREE	FREE
Meal 6	1 serving Tofu Stir-Fry (see page 300)	2	340

Week 2 Sunday			
Meal 1	2 eggs	2	150
	2 sausage links	0	134
	4 oz. V8 juice	5	23
Meal 2	½ cup cantaloupe, cubed	6	25
	½ cup cottage cheese, 1% fat	5	80
Meal 3	6-oz. chicken breast, broiled	0	186
	1 Free Foods Salad	FREE	FREE
	1 cup green beans	8	40
	1 Tbsp. Parmesan cheese, grated	0	28
Meal 4	2 oz. Havarti cheese	0	240
	4 oz. wine, rosé	6	120
Meal 5	½ banana	13	53
	8 oz. shrimp, sauteed in	0	240
	1 Tbsp. olive oil	0	120
	1 cup spinach	FREE	FREE
Meal 6	1 Curves Shake or similar protein shake (see page 59)	FREE	FREE

Week 3
Monday

Meal		Carbs	Calories
Meal 1	½ cup cottage cheese, 1% fat	5	80
	½ cup strawberries	6	23
Meal 2	1 Curves Shake or similar protein shake (see page 59)	FREE	FREE
Meal 3	1 cup carrots, cooked	11	48
	1 tsp. butter	0	34
	1 Free Foods Salad	FREE	FREE
	6 oz. ground beef, 93% lean, broiled	0	240
Meal 4	2 RyKrisp crackers	11	60
	1 serving Tuna Salad (see page 295)	3	258
Meal 5	1 cup broccoli, steamed	FREE	FREE
	1 tsp. butter	0	34
	8-oz. chicken breast, broiled	0	248
	1 Tbsp. barbeque sauce	6	25
	1 serving Creamy Coleslaw (see page 289)	3	78
Meal 6	3 oz. ham, lean	0	120
	1 oz. Havarti cheese	0	120

Week 3
Tuesday

Meal		Carbs	Calories
Meal 1	1 tsp. butter	0	34
	2 eggs	2	150
	3 oz. ham, lean	0	120
	1 piece Holland rusk dry toast	6	30
Meal 2	½ cup cantaloupe, cubed	6	25
	1 oz. cashews, roasted and salted	7	170
	½ cup cottage cheese, 1% fat	5	80
Meal 3	1 serving Greek Salad (see page 288)	6	348
Meal 4	1 Curves Shake or similar protein shake (see page 59)	FREE	FREE
Meal 5	1 cup green beans	8	40
	1 tsp. butter	0	34
	1 serving Lemony Cauliflower (see page 304)	0	75
	8 oz. orange roughy, broiled	0	216
Meal 6	1 apple, small	20	80
	1 oz. Havarti cheese	0	120

Week 3 Wednesday

Meal		Carbs	Calories
Meal 1	¼ cup blueberries	7	27
	8 oz. yogurt, plain	18	150
Meal 2	1 Curves Shake or similar protein shake (see page 59)	FREE	FREE
Meal 3	1 Free Foods Salad	FREE	FREE
	6-oz. pork chop, lean, broiled	0	225
Meal 4	1 serving Italian Soda (see page 307)	0	100
	2 oz. pistachio nuts, in shells	7	170
Meal 5	½ cup sauerkraut	FREE	FREE
	6 oz. smoked sausage, low-fat	12	330
	1 cup zucchini, sauteed in	FREE	FREE
	1 Tbsp. olive oil	0	120
Meal 6	2 oz. ham, lean	0	80
	1 oz. Havarti cheese	0	120

Week 3 Thursday

Meal		Carbs	Calories
Meal 1	2 eggs	2	150
	1 piece Holland rusk dry toast	6	30
	3 sausage links	0	200
Meal 2	2 Keebler Harvest Bakery Multigrain Crackers	11	70
	2 Tbsp. vegetable cream cheese	2	90
Meal 3	½ cup asparagus, steamed	FREE	FREE
	1 tsp. butter	0	34
	1 serving Sherry-Mushroom Chicken (see page 301)	3	288
Meal 4	1 Curves Shake or similar protein shake (see page 59)	FREE	FREE
Meal 5	1 serving Beef & Vegetable Stew (see page 296)	8	256
	1 Free Foods Salad	FREE	FREE
Meal 6	1 oz. cashews, roasted and salted	7	170
	½ cup watermelon, cubed	6	25

Week 3 Friday

Meal		Carbs	Calories
Meal 1	4 strips bacon	0	147
	2 eggs	2	150
Meal 2	1 Curves Shake or similar protein shake (see page 59)	FREE	FREE
Meal 3	1 serving Easy Frittata (see page 298)	4	325
	1 Free Foods Salad	FREE	FREE
Meal 4	1 slice bread, whole-wheat	12	70
	1 oz. cheddar cheese	0	110
	1 Tbsp. light mayonnaise	1	50
	4 oz. roast beef, deli	4	120
	1 serving Vegetable Soup (see page 291)	5	85
Meal 5	½ cup cantaloupe, cubed	6	25
	½ cup cottage cheese, 1% fat	5	80
Meal 6	2 Turkey-Lettuce Wraps (see page 293)	12	166

Week 3 Saturday

Meal		Carbs	Calories
Meal 1	1 slice bread, whole-wheat	12	70
	1 oz. Havarti cheese	0	120
	3 sausage links	0	200
Meal 2	1 Curves Shake or similar protein shake (see page 59)	FREE	FREE
Meal 3	1 serving Chicken Fajitas (see page 293)	1	280
	½ cup refried beans	25	120
Meal 4	1 oz. cashews, roasted and salted	7	170
Meal 5	5 oz. halibut, broiled	0	200
	1 serving Parmesan Vegetable Stir-Fry (see page 304)	0	175
Meal 6	1 Free Foods Salad	FREE	FREE

Week 3
Sunday

		Carbs	Calories
Meal 1	2 eggs	2	150
	3 sausage links	0	200
	8 oz. V8 juice	10	46
Meal 2	½ cup cantaloupe, cubed	6	25
	½ cup cottage cheese, 1% fat	5	80
Meal 3	6-oz. chicken breast, broiled	0	186
	1 orange, medium	16	65
	½ cup snow peas, steamed	FREE	FREE
	1 tsp. butter	0	34
Meal 4	1 oz. Havarti cheese	0	120
	4 oz. wine, rosé	6	120
Meal 5	1 Free Foods Salad	FREE	FREE
	1 cup mushrooms	FREE	FREE
	1 cup spinach	FREE	FREE
	8 oz. scallops, sauteed in	0	200
	1 Tbsp. olive oil	0	120
Meal 6	1 Curves Shake or similar protein shake (see page 59)	FREE	FREE

Week 4
Monday

		Carbs	Calories
Meal 1	½ cup cottage cheese, 1% fat	5	80
	½ cup strawberries	6	23
Meal 2	1 Curves Shake or similar protein shake (see page 59)	FREE	FREE
Meal 3	1 cup carrots, cooked	11	48
	1 tsp. butter	0	34
	6 oz. ground beef, 93% lean, broiled	0	240
	1 plum, medium	9	36
Meal 4	1 serving French Onion Soup (see page 290)	3	145
	1 Tbsp. Parmesan cheese, grated	0	28
	1 serving Italian Soda (see page 307)	0	100
Meal 5	1 cup cauliflower, steamed	FREE	FREE
	1 tsp. butter	0	34
	1 Free Foods Salad	FREE	FREE
	1 serving Spicy Chili Pork Chops (see page 302)	4	219
Meal 6	3 oz. ham, lean	0	120
	1 oz. Monterey Jack cheese	0	110
	4 oz. wine, rosé	6	120

Week 4 Tuesday

Meal	Food	Carbs	Calories
Meal 1	2 eggs	2	150
	1 tsp. butter	0	34
	2 oz. ham, lean	0	80
Meal 2	½ cup cantaloupe, cubed	6	25
	½ cup cottage cheese, 1% fat	5	80
Meal 3	1 serving Greek Salad (see page 288)	6	348
Meal 4	1 Curves Shake or similar protein shake (see page 59)	FREE	FREE
Meal 5	½ cup corn, whole-kernel	13	66
	1 serving Jamaican Seafood Medley (see page 299)	6	283
	1 cup zucchini, sauteed in	FREE	FREE
	1 Tbsp. olive oil	0	120
Meal 6	2 oz. cheddar cheese	0	220
	1 serving Frozen Chocolate Mousse (see page 306)	9	127
	2 Keebler Harvest Bakery Multigrain Crackers	11	70

Week 4 Wednesday

Meal	Food	Carbs	Calories
Meal 1	¼ cup blueberries	7	27
	8 oz. yogurt, plain	18	150
Meal 2	1 Curves Shake or similar protein shake (see page 59)	FREE	FREE
Meal 3	6-oz. pork chop, lean, broiled	0	225
	½ cup sauerkraut	FREE	FREE
	½ cup red bell pepper	FREE	FREE
	½ cup zucchini, sauteed in	FREE	FREE
	1 Tbsp. olive oil	0	120
Meal 4	1 serving Italian Stuffed Mushrooms (see page 294)	13	177
	8 oz. V8 juice	10	46
Meal 5	1 serving Beef Tenderloin with Blue Cheese (see page 297)	1	383
	1 Free Foods Salad	FREE	FREE
Meal 6	3 oz. ham, lean	0	120
	1 oz. Monterey Jack cheese	0	110

Week 4 Thursday		Carbs	Calories
Meal 1	2 eggs	2	150
	1 piece Holland rusk dry toast	6	30
	3 sausage links	0	200
Meal 2	2 Keebler Harvest Bakery Multigrain Crackers	11	70
	2 Tbsp. vegetable cream cheese	2	90
	1 cup watermelon, cubed	12	50
Meal 3	1 cup broccoli, steamed	FREE	FREE
	1 tsp. butter	0	34
	6-oz. chicken breast, broiled	0	186
Meal 4	1 Curves Shake or similar protein shake (see page 59)	FREE	FREE
Meal 5	1 serving Beef & Vegetable Stew (see page 296)	8	256
	1 Free Foods Salad	FREE	FREE
Meal 6	1 oz. cheddar cheese	0	110
	1 oz. peanuts, dry-roasted	5	160

Week 4 Friday			
Meal 1	1 tsp. butter	0	34
	2 eggs	2	150
	3 oz. ham, lean	0	120
Meal 2	1 Curves Shake or similar protein shake (see page 59)	FREE	FREE
Meal 3	½ cup strawberries	6	23
	2 Turkey-Lettuce Wraps (see page 293)	12	166
Meal 4	2 oz. cheddar cheese	0	220
	2 RyKrisp crackers	11	60
Meal 5	1 cup asparagus	FREE	FREE
	1 tsp. butter	0	34
	1 Free Foods Salad	FREE	FREE
	8-oz. tuna steak (fresh), marinated in	0	247
	Seafood Marinade (see page 301)	2	30
Meal 6	½ cantaloupe, cubed	6	25
	½ cup cottage cheese, 1% fat	5	80

Week 4 Saturday

		Carbs	Calories
Meal 1	1 slice bread, whole-wheat	12	70
	1 oz. Monterey Jack cheese	0	110
	3 sausage links	0	200
Meal 2	1 Curves Shake or similar protein shake (see page 59)	FREE	FREE
Meal 3	1 oz. cheddar cheese	0	110
	4 oz. ground beef, 93% lean, broiled	0	160
	½ cup refried beans	25	120
	2 Tbsp. salsa	2	10
Meal 4	4 oz. salmon, broiled	0	207
	1 serving Spicy Zucchini Boats (see page 305)	2	195
Meal 5	1 Free Foods Salad	FREE	FREE
Meal 6	1 oz. peanuts, dry-roasted	5	160

Week 4 Sunday

Meal 1	4 strips bacon	0	147
	1 egg	1	75
Meal 2	½ cup cantaloupe, cubed	6	25
	½ cup cottage cheese, 1% fat	5	80
Meal 3	1 apple, small	20	80
	6-oz. chicken breast, broiled	0	186
	½ cup snow peas, steamed	FREE	FREE
	1 tsp. butter	0	34
Meal 4	2 oz. Monterey Jack cheese	0	220
	2 RyKrisp crackers	11	60
	4 oz. wine, rosé	6	120
Meal 5	1 Free Foods Salad	FREE	FREE
	1 cup mushrooms	FREE	FREE
	1 cup spinach	FREE	FREE
	8 oz. orange roughy, sauteed in	0	216
	1 Tbsp. olive oil	0	120
Meal 6	1 Curves Shake or similar protein shake (see page 59)	FREE	FREE

Week 5 Monday		Carbs	Calories
Meal 1	1 slice bread, whole-wheat	12	70
	1 Tbsp. light mayonnaise	1	50
	1 oz. Swiss cheese	0	110
	2 oz. turkey breast, deli	2	60
Meal 2	½ cup baby carrots	5	24
	½ cup cottage cheese, 1% fat	5	80
Meal 3	1 serving French Onion Soup (see page 290)	3	145
	6 oz. ground beef, 93% lean, broiled	0	240
Meal 4	½ cup grapes, seedless	14	57
	1 oz. macadamia nuts	5	160
Meal 5	1 cup broccoli, steamed	FREE	FREE
	1 tsp. butter	0	34
	1 Free Foods Salad	FREE	FREE
	1 serving Spicy Chili Pork Chops (see page 302)	4	219
Meal 6	1 Curves Shake or similar protein shake (see page 59)	FREE	FREE

Week 5 Tuesday			
Meal 1	2 eggs	2	150
	2 oz. ham, lean	0	80
Meal 2	½ cup cottage cheese, 1% fat	5	80
	½ cup strawberries	6	23
Meal 3	1 slice bread, whole-wheat	12	70
	½ Tbsp. butter	0	51
	6-oz. chicken breast, broiled	0	186
	1 serving Spinach Salad with Orange Vinaigrette (see page 288)	3	101
Meal 4	1 Curves Shake or similar protein shake (see page 59)	FREE	FREE
Meal 5	1 serving Frozen Chocolate Mousse (see page 306)	9	127
	1 serving Jamaican Seafood Medley (see page 299)	6	283
	1 cup zucchini, sauteed in	FREE	FREE
	1 Tbsp. olive oil	0	120
Meal 6	1 oz. almonds, roasted and salted	4	180
	1 oz. cheddar cheese	0	110
	1 peach, medium, peeled	9	37

Week 5 Wednesday

Meal		Carbs	Calories
Meal 1	1 medium peach	9	37
	4 oz. yogurt, plain	9	75
Meal 2	1 Curves Shake or similar protein shake (see page 59)	FREE	FREE
Meal 3	1 oz. cheddar cheese	0	110
	6 oz. ground beef, 93% lean, broiled	0	240
	½ cup refried beans	25	120
	2 Tbsp. salsa	2	10
Meal 4	1 serving Spicy Zucchini Boats (see page 305)	2	195
	1 serving Vegetable Soup (see page 291)	5	85
Meal 5	1 Free Foods Salad	FREE	FREE
	8-oz. pork chop, lean, broiled	0	225
Meal 6	2 oz. roast beef, deli	2	60
	1 oz. Swiss cheese	0	110

Week 5 Thursday

Meal		Carbs	Calories
Meal 1	4 strips bacon	0	147
	2 eggs	2	150
Meal 2	2 Keebler Harvest Bakery Multigrain Crackers	11	70
	2 Tbsp. vegetable cream cheese	2	90
	1 cup watermelon, cubed	12	50
Meal 3	6-oz. chicken breast, broiled	0	186
	1 Tbsp. blue cheese	0	47
	½ cup peas, green, steamed	11	60
	1 tsp. butter	0	34
Meal 4	1 Curves Shake or similar protein shake (see page 59)	FREE	FREE
Meal 5	1 Free Foods Salad	FREE	FREE
	6-oz. sirloin steak, broiled	0	323
Meal 6	1 oz. cheddar cheese	0	110
	4 oz. wine, rosé	6	120

Week 5 Friday		Carbs	Calories
Meal 1	1 egg	1	75
	1 piece Holland rusk dry toast	6	30
	3 sausage links	0	200
Meal 2	1 Curves Shake or similar protein shake (see page 59)	FREE	FREE
Meal 3	1 serving Creamy Coleslaw (see page 289)	3	78
	4 oz. ground beef, 93% lean, broiled	0	160
	1 Tbsp. barbeque sauce	6	25
Meal 4	1 serving Italian Stuffed Mushrooms (see page 294)	13	177
Meal 5	1 Free Foods Salad	FREE	FREE
	1 serving Lemony Cauliflower (see page 304)	0	75
	8 oz. shrimp, sauteed in	0	240
	1 Tbsp. olive oil	0	120
Meal 6	½ cup cottage cheese, 1% fat	5	80
	½ cup strawberries	6	23

Week 5 Saturday			
Meal 1	1 slice bread, whole-wheat	12	70
	1 oz. cheddar cheese	0	110
	3 sausage links	0	200
Meal 2	1 Curves Shake or similar protein shake (see page 59)	FREE	FREE
Meal 3	1 Free Foods Salad	FREE	FREE
Meal 4	6-oz. chicken breast, broiled	0	186
	½ cup snow peas, steamed	FREE	FREE
	1 tsp. butter	0	34
Meal 5	1 serving Chinese Vegetables (see page 303)	8	160
	8 oz. red snapper, broiled	0	226
Meal 6	½ cup French vanilla ice cream	15	160
	1 oz. peanuts, dry-roasted	5	160
	½ cup strawberries	6	23

Week 5 Sunday		Carbs	Calories
Meal 1	4 strips bacon	0	147
	2 eggs	2	150
Meal 2	½ cup cottage cheese, 1% fat	5	80
	½ cup watermelon, cubed	6	25
Meal 3	1 cup green beans	8	40
	1 tsp. butter	0	34
	½ cup sauerkraut	FREE	FREE
	8 oz. smoked sausage, low-fat	16	440
Meal 4	2 Keebler Harvest Bakery Multigrain Crackers	11	70
	1 oz. Swiss cheese	0	110
Meal 5	1 Free Foods Salad	FREE	FREE
	1 serving Sherry-Mushroom Chicken (see page 301)	3	288
Meal 6	1 Curves Shake or similar protein shake (see page 59)	FREE	FREE

Curves Profile

PEGGY D.

ANCHORAGE, ALASKA

Curves literally saved my life. Before I joined Curves, I weighed 300 pounds and wore a size 26. Size 10 is *loose* on me now. I was a chunky kid. I slimmed down a bit in high school, but after I married and started having kids, I began putting on more pounds, and it just escalated from there. My blood pressure became sky-high, and my doctor told me that the only way to deal with my blood pressure problem was to go on a diet, start exercising, and take medication to lower it. I had already been on every diet known to man. I had my stomach stapled 20-something years ago, and that didn't work.

I tried acupuncture—I did it all and nothing worked. The one thing I had never tried before was exercise. I realized that if I didn't do something about my weight, I would probably die young. I wouldn't be around to see my grandchildren grow up or to be able to do all the things that my husband and I wanted to do together now that the kids were grown. I also had another important reason to lose weight: My husband and I have a cabin in the woods where we love to go, and he flies his own small plane to get there. I always felt very uncomfortable in the plane, and I was afraid that we might crash because of my weight. This may sound silly, but weight and balance are very important in a small airplane. All of this played a part in my decision to go to Curves. I woke on a Friday morning—I remember the exact date: February 9, 2001—and I decided I was just sick and tired of being the way I was. A friend of mine had told me about the Permanent Weight Loss Without Permanent Dieting program being offered at Curves, and that kind of sparked my interest. I really liked the part about "without permanent dieting." I started following the meal plan first, but I still didn't want to exercise. Two months later, I was 30 pounds lighter! I decided that Gary Heavin knew what he was talking about and I would at least give the exercise program a try. In

April 2001, I officially joined Curves. I met a great group of women, and I was really surprised at how much I enjoyed going. It was tough at first, but the more I worked out, the easier it became and the faster the weight came off. Working out made it a lot easier to stick with my weight-management program. The real joy of this program is that it's only a half-hour workout. You don't get bored because you don't stay on a machine for more than 30 seconds at a time. Thirty minutes and you're done. Anybody can do that! You feel good about yourself, and you feel great because you've had such a terrific workout. And I'm healthier than I've been in years. My blood pressure is normal, and I don't need to take any medication.

I tell everybody I can about Curves. My advice to anyone who has to lose a lot of weight is never give up, and give Curves a try.

CHAPTER 7

NUTRITION FOR A GREAT BODY

We use food to celebrate holidays, reward good behavior ("I just walked two miles; I can have that ice cream cone!"), stave off boredom, relieve stress, soothe hurt feelings, and elevate mood. Nature had something else in mind. The primary function of food is to provide energy to fuel all body functions, from walking to thinking to the beating of your heart to the maintenance and repair of your cells. Nature did not anticipate the recreational eating common in the 21st century!

Our primitive ancestors, who were typically strong and lean, may have stayed that way because they had few choices. These hunter-gatherers ate whatever they could find in the wild and did not go home to pantries and refrigerators packed with sugar-laden snacks, soda, and assorted junk food.

Even our more immediate ancestors were not bombarded with the dizzying array of food that we have today. In the early 20th century, the typical local grocery store stocked a few dozen staple items; today there are *50,000* different varieties of food sold in supermarkets. More isn't necessarily better—most of these new foods are pure, unadulterated junk. There's row upon row of chips, highly sugared cereals masquerading as breakfast, and endless amounts of snack food. Moreover, on every block, in every small town and big city, you will find a fast-food restaurant selling high-fat, high-calorie, high-carbohydrate "supersized" meals.

The real problem today is that food is abundant and easily available. Unlike our primitive ancestors, whose survival depended on their ability to find enough food so they wouldn't starve, our survival depends on our ability to become discriminating food consumers. In this chapter, I will give you the tools you will need to make good food choices, whether you eat at home, at work, in the front seat of your car, or in any restaurant. Armed with this information, you can shop wisely and well at any supermarket, order a perfectly acceptable meal at any fast-food restaurant, and always have the right food on hand wherever you go. You will have the knowledge—and the power—to eat well.

Know Your Nutrients

There are two types of nutrients: macronutrients and micronutrients. Macronutrients—protein, fat, and carbohydrates—provide us with energy. Micronutrients are the vitamins and minerals that are required to run the body, but they are consumed in relatively small quantities. Without micronutrients, macronutrients could not be broken down and utilized by the body. (For more information on vitamins, read Chapter 11.) We need both macronutrients and micronutrients to survive.

Protein

CALORIES: 4 per gram

BEST SOURCES: Lean meat, skinless poultry, most fish, eggs, low-fat and no-fat dairy products

FACTS: There are 7 grams of usable protein per ounce of lean meat, poultry, and fish.

Women need a *minimum* of 50 to 100 grams of protein daily and more if they are working out regularly.

> If you don't eat enough protein when you are on a weight-loss diet, you will lose muscle and get flabby.
>
> As women age, it becomes more difficult to absorb protein from food.

The word "protein" dates back to the ancient Greek word *protos,* which means "first." The ancient Greeks got it right! Protein is a vitally important nutrient; it is literally the stuff from which we are made. During digestion, protein is broken down into smaller units called amino acids, which combine in different ways to form the various cells and tissues of the body. Amino acids also provide energy if the body needs it, but unlike carbohydrates, they do not produce a spike in insulin.

There are 22 different amino acids. Fourteen of these can be made by the body and are called "nonessential" amino acids. The other eight amino acids can be obtained only through food and are called "essential" amino acids. Protein is found in both animals and plants. Protein derived from animal products, meat, eggs, and dairy products contains all eight essential amino acids; these foods are complete protein sources. Only a handful of plant foods have all eight essential amino acids— these include soybeans and soy foods. Most plant sources of protein, such as legumes (beans) and nuts, contain some but not all of the essential amino acids. If you do not eat animal products, you can compensate for the shortfall by combining complementary proteins. For example, amino acids that are missing in rice can be found in beans; therefore, a dish of rice and beans will give you all eight essential amino acids. Obviously, it takes more careful planning for vegetarians to get their full complement of amino acids, but it can be done.

Our prehistoric ancestors thrived on a diet of 30 percent protein— that's about three times the amount most women eat today. The U.S. government's Daily Value (DV) for protein for women is a mere 50 grams, and many women do not consume even this meager amount.

Here's the most damning evidence of all against the low-protein, high-carbohydrate diet: Do you know how archaeologists determine whether people of a prehistoric society were hunters or farmers? They examine the teeth and bone remains. If the bones are dense and strong, and the teeth are not decayed, they know that they have found a community of hunter-gatherers, which means they ate a high-protein diet. If, on the other hand, the bones are frail and underdeveloped, and the teeth are decayed, they know they have located a community of agriculturists—that is, carbohydrate eaters. What does that tell you about protein diets versus carbohydrate diets?

Women over age 50 take note: Even if you are eating ample amounts of protein, your body may not be absorbing it well. Proteins are tough to digest—think about it: A piece of meat is harder to chew than a piece of bread. In the stomach, hydrochloric acid (HCl) and pepsin, a digestive enzyme, work together to break down proteins in the stomach. The problem is, as we age, as many as half of all people over age 60 may have hypochlorydia, a condition in which the stomach doesn't produce enough HCl. Hypochlorydia is particularly common among women, who may need to eat even more protein to get adequate absorption. (You can also take digestive enzymes to promote better protein absorption.) The problem is, the symptoms of low HCl are the same as indigestion, which people often treat by taking antacids, which only further reduce HCl levels and aggravate symptoms. If you have indigestion, be sure to check with your doctor about hypochlorydia before popping an antacid pill.

Fat

CALORIES: 9 per gram

BEST SOURCES: Olive oil, omega-3 fatty acids, butter (not margarine)

FACTS: Fat calories add up quickly. Use added fat sparingly. Omega-3 fatty acids found in fish are essential for good physical and mental health.

Avoid processed, baked products and fried foods containing trans-fatty acids (french fries, snack foods, chips, etc.).

Beware of fake fats (such as olestra).

Considering the fat phobia in the United States, you would think that fat is a useless, unhealthy nutrient that the world would be better off without. Nothing could be further from the truth. Dietary fat is essential for a healthy body. It provides the raw material for cholesterol, which is made into hormones and is the structure of cell membranes, the protective covering around all cells. Fat is necessary for the absorption of the fat-soluble vitamins: A, D, E, and K. Your brain contains a high concentration of fat. If you don't eat enough fat, your skin will dry out and your hair and nails will get brittle, as often happens to people on very low-calorie, low-fat diets.

Not all fats are the same. There are many different types of fat in the food we eat, and some are better for you than others.

Essential Fatty Acids

Essential fatty acids are the Cadillacs of fat. Your body needs them, but it can't make them, so they must be obtained through food. There are two types of essential fatty acids: omega-6 and omega-3. We get ample amounts of omega-6 fats from nuts, vegetable oils, and grains, but many of us are lacking in omega-3 fats, which are found primarily in fatty fish, such as salmon, mackerel, flounder, albacore tuna, and sardines. If you don't get enough omega-3 fats in your diet, your health will suffer, especially your mental health. Low levels of omega-3 fats in the diet have been linked to depression, a problem that affects about 25 percent of all women at some point in their lives. If you are prone to depression, it's very important to get enough omega-3 fatty acids in your diet.

Butter Versus Margarine

Much of the fats consumed in the United States are saturated fats from dairy products, meat, and poultry. Peanut butter and coconut are rare breeds among vegetables, because they contain a sizable amount of saturated fat. Saturated fats are solid at room temperature. Fats from vegetable sources—polyunsaturated fats—are liquid at room temperature. When it comes to fat, once again the conventional wisdom has let us down. After World War II, the nutritional experts told us to give up butter (a saturated fat) in favor of margarine (a polyunsaturated fat) because saturated fat promoted heart disease. It's true that in some people, eating a diet rich in saturated fat will elevate blood-cholesterol levels. Ironically, it now appears that margarine is even more harmful.

In 1995, a landmark study involving more than 80,000 women, the Harvard Nurses' Study, showed that nurses who ate margarine had a higher incidence of cardiovascular disease than those who ate butter! The medical community was shocked at the results, but those of us who knew something about nutrition were not. Polyunsaturated fat is unstable, so it creates a higher potential for free radicals, chemicals that are manufactured in our bodies as a product of normal energy production. Free radicals are very unstable oxygen molecules. When they bind with healthy cells—that is, when the molecules in the cells become oxidized—they give off energy and cause a great deal of damage. Free radicals also promote the formation of plaque, an accumulation of cholesterol and other cells that clogs arteries and can trigger a heart attack. Why is butter better? Butter is a very stable compound and is not easily oxidized, and it will not become a free-radical magnet in your body. That's why it's better to eat moderate amounts of butter instead of margarine. (I say "moderate" because butter is very fattening.)

There's yet another reason to avoid most brands of margarine and vegetable oils: Some polyunsaturated oils and margarine undergo a process called "hydrogenation" to make them useful for baking and to extend their shelf life. This process creates a dangerous type of fat called "trans-fatty acids." Trans-fatty acids become incorporated into your cell membranes and make them rigid, which can interfere with normal cell function. These fats have been linked to a pre-diabetic condition called "insulin resistance" and can raise blood-cholesterol and triglyceride levels. (Triglycerides are a type of lipid that, in excess, can increase your risk of heart disease.) The problem is that trans-fats are a common ingredient in processed baked goods, chips, and other junk foods and fried foods. Recently, some food manufacturers have removed trans-fats from their products and labeled them as such. There are even some brands of margarine that do not contain trans-fats. But unless a label clearly states "No Trans-Fatty Acids," you can assume that they are present in most processed and fried foods, and most brands of margarine.

My Choice Is Olive Oil

I personally don't eat butter or margarine. My fat of choice is olive oil, a monounsaturated fat that is stable—so it resists free-radical attack—and delicious. It is a staple of the Mediterranean diet. In fact, in Italy, where they consume huge quantities of olive oil, they have one of the lowest rates of cardiovascular disease on the planet. I cook my eggs in olive oil, I dip my bread in olive oil, and I recommend that you get into the olive oil habit too!

Forgo the Fake Fats

I'm not a big fan of fake fats, such as olestra, the artificial, nondigestible fat that is used in snack foods. If consumed in high enough doses, these fats may wash fat-soluble vitamins out of your body, in addition to causing abdominal cramping and gastrointestinal distress in some people. Keep in mind that low-fat or no-fat snack foods still contain high amounts of carbohydrates, which are converted into sugar and which end up being stored as fat anyway!

Carbohydrates

CALORIES: 4 per gram

BEST SOURCES: Fresh vegetables and low-sugar fruits (melon, berries, cherries), whole, unprocessed grains

FACTS: Carbohydrates are broken down into sugar during digestion.

Carbohydrates include a wide array of foods, from brownies to broccoli to beans.

The wrong carbohydrates can be addicting and have a disastrous effect on your metabolism, your mood, and your weight.

Carbohydrates encompass a wide variety of foods, ranging from grains to vegetables to fruits to legumes. All carbohydrates are converted into glucose, or sugar, the form in which your body can utilize them. The brain reacts to the sugar rush by telling the pancreas to produce insulin, the hormone that allows your body to use sugar but also promotes fat storage. It's not just sweets, like cookies and cakes, that are a problem— starchy carbohydrates like bread, rice, potatoes, and pasta can be just as troublesome. These foods are broken down very rapidly in the blood-stream, causing a sharp rise in blood-sugar levels followed by the in-evitable steep drop, leaving you feeling tired, depleted, and starving for more high-sugar carbohydrates! As I discussed in Chapter 2, the car-bohydrate sugar high is highly addictive, and most people need to be careful about their carbohydrate intake. There are good carbohydrates and bad carbohydrates, and if you want to stay slim, you have to know the difference.

Carbohydrates are divided into two groups: refined and complex. Re-fined carbohydrates include soda, candy, and the processed white flour and grain products (white bread, cookies, pasta, and most commercial ce-reals) that have been stripped of their vitamins and minerals. Ironically, the mineral chromium, typically depleted from wheat products during the refining process, actually helps the body regulate blood sugar! Refined carbohydrates are also missing another key ingredient—fiber, an indi-gestible nutrient found in plants, which also has a stabilizing influence on blood-sugar levels. Fiber slows down the absorption and breakdown of carbohydrates in the body, thereby preventing sharp sugar surges. Unfor-tunately, fiber can also shorten the shelf life of food, so manufacturers simply remove it. Without fiber, refined carbohydrates are little better than pure table sugar.

Choose Slow-Burning Carbohydrates

Complex carbohydrates (fruits, vegetables, legumes, and whole grains) contain significant amounts of fiber. In moderate amounts, these are healthy foods to incorporate into a normal diet. I know that according to the government Food Guide Pyramid, you're supposed to eat 6 to 11 servings of grains every day, but even whole grains are relatively high in sugar, and if you gorge on them, you will be back in diet hell before you know it. If you eat grains along with some protein and fat, the other foods will slow the breakdown and absorption of the carbohydrates, and that will help reduce the blood-sugar surge.

Most fruits and grains contain considerably more natural sugar than vegetables do. Therefore, with few exceptions, vegetables are your best source of carbohydrates, especially the leafy green variety, for example, broccoli, lettuce, celery, escarole, and brussels sprouts (see the Free Foods list, page 57). You will notice that the Free Foods list consists of a wide variety of low-carbohydrate vegetables. (You can eat unlimited quantities of Free Foods without counting them in your daily total carbohydrate allowance, which is why the carbs in Free Food ingredients don't count toward the total carbs for the recipes in the back of the book.)

Fruit Is Not a Free Food

Some fruits are better for you than others. Berries, melon, and red plums are good fruit choices because they don't produce as high a sugar spike as do sweeter fruits like pineapples, grapes, and oranges, because berries, melon, and red plums are lower in carbohydrates. Avoid fruit juice—it contains all the sugar of fruit without the beneficial fiber. You can check out the carbohydrate content of common fruits on pages 65–66.

True carbohydrate addicts will do much better on diets if they restrict their intake of starchy and sweet carbohydrates. *The only way to stop carbohydrate cravings is to not eat carbohydrates.* Stick to the acceptable vegetables, forgo all grains, and limit your intake of fruit while you are on Phase 1 and Phase 2.

Fiber

- Few Americans consume enough fiber.
- Eat about 30 grams of fiber daily.
- Eating fiber-rich foods can help keep you slim.
- Unsweetened bran cereals (Fiber One has 6.5 grams of fiber per ¼ cup; All-Bran has 5 grams of fiber per ¼ cup) are great sources of fiber.

Fiber refers to food substances found in plants that are not digested or absorbed by the body. It's described as a nonnutrient because we discard it, yet it's of vital importance. Numerous studies have linked a high-fiber diet to a decreased risk of chronic diseases such as diabetes, heart disease, and nearly all gastrointestinal problems.

There are two types of fiber: soluble and insoluble (also known as roughage). Think of soluble and insoluble fiber as the yin and yang of nutrition. They are exact opposites, yet they are meant to work together.

Soluble fiber is found in foods such as apples, oat bran, lentils, barley, and broccoli. Soluble fiber forms a gel-like substance that expands and slows down the movement of food through the stomach and upper digestive system. Eating foods rich in soluble fiber will make you feel full and more satisfied. In addition, soluble fiber is very effective at lowering blood-cholesterol levels.

Insoluble fiber is found in foods such as celery, fresh greens, wheat bran, and legumes like kidney and pinto beans. It speeds up the movement of food through the intestines, where you want it to be speeded up. This not only prevents constipation but also reduces the exposure of the gut to toxins that are normally found in food and that may increase the risk of developing certain kinds of cancers. In addition, insoluble fiber may prevent the absorption of some calories, which is a good thing if you're trying to lose weight. Type II diabetics are often told to eat more fiber because it slows down the absorption of sugar, preventing a spike in insulin. As far as I'm concerned, this is good advice for everyone.

The fiber content in commonly consumed foods such as bread and cereal varies from brand to brand. Be sure to choose the products with the highest amount of fiber. Read food labels! You will see that some whole-grain breads have four to five grams of fiber per slice, whereas white Italian bread barely has one gram. If you choose the right bread, you can include eight to ten grams of fiber in your sandwich. If you add vegetables like peppers, onions, sprouts, and lettuce to your sandwich (all Free Foods), you can add a few extra fiber grams to your daily intake.

If you are used to getting your fiber from grains and you are on the Carbohydrate-Sensitive Plan, you may be eating less fiber than normal, especially if you're in Phase 1, during which you must limit your carbohydrate intake to 20 grams daily. You can easily make up the difference by filling your plate with Free Foods, which are packed with fiber. Try to eat at least 5 cups of Free Foods daily. That will give you an additional 12 or so fiber grams. Powdered fiber (such as Metamucil) can be added to your Curves Shake or other protein shake, or to yogurt, to boost your fiber intake. If you use a fiber supplement, be sure to drink plenty of water to avoid digestive distress.

Water

- Drink eight 8-ounce glasses of water daily.
- If you are on the higher protein, Carbohydrate-Sensitive Plan, you *must* be vigilant about drinking enough water.
- Caffeinated beverages are mild diuretics—they don't count as water.
- Water is the *best* beverage. Mineral water and seltzer are fine.

More than half your body consists of water, and you need to replenish it constantly. Water is essential for normal digestion and proper temperature control, and it creates the necessary environment for the chemical reactions that make up the body's metabolism and sustain life. Water also protects the kidneys and helps detoxify the body.

Water not only helps you feel your best, it also helps you look your best. From midlife on, cells tend to lose their moisture content, which can cause skin to become flatter and drier, and facial lines and wrinkles to become more prominent. Keeping your skin cells well hydrated will give them a more youthful, healthy look.

If you are consuming high amounts of protein, you must drink enough water to prevent the buildup of ketones. (See page 50.) If you are not willing to do this, you should not be on a high-protein diet.

What about other beverages? Fruit juice and regular soda are high in sugar and are not great choices, at least while you are on Phase 1 and Phase 2. The average glass of soda or sweetened tea has about 150 calories and 40 grams of carbohydrates. Sugar-free beverages are okay in limited consumption, but they are filled with chemicals and are no substitute for your eight glasses of water. No-calorie seltzer is fine, and since it is basically water with some bubbles, you can use it interchangeably with water. Bottled water from a reputable distributor is great if it's in your budget or if you are worried about the water quality in your area, but it's not necessary. Costco offers bottled water in volume at steep discounts, and so do many of the larger supermarket chains. There are also several water-purification systems on the market that can be used at home to improve the quality of tap water, ranging from inexpensive pitchers with disposable filters that clean chemicals and impurities to more elaborate home filtration systems.

Salt

At one time, the standard advice regarding salt use was "Don't!" It was believed that if you ate too much salt, it could cause high blood pressure. We now know that excess salt consumption is only a problem for people who are salt-sensitive. About 26 percent of people with normal blood pressure and 58 percent of those with high blood pressure are believed to be salt-sensitive—that is, eating salt will raise their blood pressure. For everyone else, salt is fine. In fact, salt is not bad. It is composed mainly of sodium, which is a basic component of blood. Sodium raises blood pressure by increasing the volume of fluid in the body. The more fluid there is to pump, the harder the heart has to work. The key is to maintain the right salt-to-water ratio in the body. At times, too little salt can be a problem. I remember reading about a heat wave in California a few years ago, during which elderly people on self-imposed salt-restriction diets were dying from dehydration because they didn't eat enough salt!

How do you know if you are salt-sensitive? If you already have high blood pressure, you can try reducing your salt intake and see if your blood pressure goes down. If it doesn't go down within a week or so, it's a sign that you are not salt-sensitive. If you don't have high blood pressure but feel bloated or swollen after a salty meal, that could be a sign that salt is your problem. If you are elderly, African-American, or have an immediate relative who is salt-sensitive, you have a greater risk of being salt-sensitive.

If you are salt-sensitive, you should not eat more than 2,400 milligrams of sodium daily. Since there is naturally occurring sodium in most foods, you cannot use added salt if you want to limit your salt intake. Please keep in mind that there is a great deal of salt in processed foods such as frozen dinners, canned soups, and snack foods, and if you have a problem with salt, you should avoid processed food as much as possible or buy low-sodium brands.

If you need to cut back on sodium, you can try one of the potassium-based salts sold at health-food stores. If you have a heart condition, check with your doctor before using these products.

If you hate the bitter taste of cruciferous vegetables (like broccoli) but love their health benefits, try sprinkling a small amount of salt on them. It will make them taste sweeter.

Artificial Sweeteners—The Lesser of Two Evils

I'm not a big fan of artificial sweeteners (I'm not a big fan of artificial anything), but I understand that they can be an important tool for dieters. If you have a lot of weight to lose and drinking diet soda or using an artificial sweetener in your coffee helps you stay the course, then I say by all means use it. We even include a recipe here for a chocolate mousse that uses sucralose (Splenda), a new artificial sweetener, instead of sugar. I understand the need to taste something sweet once in a while, especially when you are denying yourself many of the foods that you love, but when you have gotten down to your desired weight, I recommend that you try to eliminate artificial sweeteners from your diet as much as possible.

Some people may have an adverse reaction to artificial sweeteners, particularly aspartame, and may experience dizziness, headaches, and stomachaches, and just feel jittery. In rare cases, the use of artificial sweeteners may lead to more severe side effects, including neurological problems for susceptible people. In fact, some scientists believe that aspartame is a nerve toxin—that is, it can overexcite and kill brain cells and may increase the risk of Alzheimer's disease and Parkinson's disease. This is very controversial and not accepted by mainstream nutritionists, but I mention it because if you are at increased risk of developing these problems, you may want to avoid aspartame. Obviously, if you suspect that you may be experiencing any untoward symptoms after using these products, discontinue using them.

Alcohol

Alcoholic beverages are metabolized as sugar and are counted as carbohydrates in Phase 1 and Phase 2 of both diet plans. Due to the fact that they are loaded with calories, I don't recommend drinking any alcoholic beverages during Phase 1 of either the Calorie-Sensitive or the Carbohydrate-Sensitive Meal Plan. In Phase 2, you can have an occasional drink (one or two per week), but do keep track of both calories and carbohydrate content. For example, a regular 12-ounce serving of beer contains about 160 calories and 8 to 10 carbohydrate grams. A light beer has 100 calories and 3.5 to 7 carbohydrate grams. A 3.5-ounce glass of wine has 70 calories and up to 2 carbohydrate grams. Sweetened mixed drinks should be avoided. Depending on how it's made, a whiskey sour can contain 160 calories and 14 grams of carbohydrates—considering that your total for Phase 2 is 60 grams of carbohydrates daily, even one mixed drink can take a bite out of your carbohydrate allowance.

When you are in Phase 3, a glass of wine or beer with dinner, and even an occasional mixed drink, is fine and may even be beneficial, as long as you do not have a problem with alcohol. (And please don't drink and drive.)

Drinking more than two alcoholic beverages daily for men, or more than one alcoholic beverage daily for women, increases the risk of developing many different diseases, including heart disease and some forms of cancer. Alcohol boosts estrogen levels in women, which may promote the growth of estrogen-sensitive tumors. If you are at high risk for developing breast cancer, you should drink alcohol sparingly, if at all.

Phytochemicals

On the Curves Meal Plan, many of you will be eating more vegetables and fruit than you have in your entire life. At the same time you are slimming down, you are also filling your body with important disease-fighting compounds called "phytochemicals," which are abundant in fruits and vegetables. If you haven't been eating a wide variety of vegetables and fruits, you are losing out on nature's best form of preventive medicine. Many phytochemicals are antioxidants, which neutralize the negative effects of free radicals, which are highly unstable chemicals made in our bodies during energy production. Free radicals can damage healthy cells and tissues, and have been linked to nearly every serious ailment, from heart disease to neurological problems to cancer and premature aging. Did you know that free radicals can even cause your skin to wrinkle?

Several vitamins and minerals, such as vitamins C and E, and zinc, are important antioxidants and often work in tandem with phytochemicals to keep free radicals in check. There are literally thousands of phytochemicals, and only a handful have actually been studied for their disease-fighting potential. Most phytochemicals can be found in the pigments of plants—for example, dark green leafy vegetables have different phytochemicals than yellow and orange vegetables do. You need to eat an assortment of brightly colored fruits and vegetables daily to make sure that you are getting a full range of phytochemicals. Here is a small sample of some of the important phytochemicals in food.

Anthocyanins: Found in blueberries and bilberries, anthocyanins are potent antioxidants that appear to be important for good eyesight, especially night vision. They may also make you look and feel younger. In a recent study conducted by USDA researchers, rats that were fed blueberries showed fewer signs of mental or physical aging than those that were not.

Carotenoids: Found in orange and yellow fruits and vegetables, and in green leafy vegetables, there are more than 60 carotenoids in food, including the most famous, beta carotene, which is converted into vitamin A in the body. Carotenoids boost immune function and may reduce your risk of developing certain forms of cancer. Two carotenoids, lutein and zeaxanthin, found in raw spinach and kale, can help preserve vision and may decrease the risk of macular degeneration, the leading cause of blindness among people over age 50. Another carotenoid, lycopene, found in red peppers, tomatoes, and ruby red grapefruits, may protect against cervical cancer in women and prostate cancer in men. (Cooked tomatoes are the best source.)

Ellagic acid: Strawberries and cherries are loaded with ellagic acid, a natural antioxidant that is believed to be a potent cancer fighter.

Flavonoids: Found in tea, oranges, citrus fruits, apples, and onions, among other foods, these amazing phytochemicals work with vitamin C in the body to control free radicals, enhance immune function, and prevent the oxidation of LDL, or "bad" cholesterol, which can increase the risk of heart disease.

Indole-c-carbinole: Found in broccoli, cauliflower, kale, cabbage, and brussels sprouts (*all Free Foods!*), this phytochemical deactivates potent estrogens in the body that can stimulate the growth of estrogen-sensitive cells, particularly those that could promote breast cancer.

Isoflavone: Isoflavone is a type of flavonoid found in soy foods. In the body, it is converted into phytoestrogens, very weak estrogenlike compounds that may block the action of stronger estrogens that can promote breast cancer in women and prostate cancer in men. Due to their estrogenic activity, isoflavones may also help relieve menopausal symptoms such as hot flashes and insomnia, and can be used by women as an alternative to hormone-replacement therapy. (See page 234.)

Quercetin: A member of the bioflavonoid family found in onions, apples, and garlic, quercetin helps reduce inflammation and may relieve allergic symptoms.

Sulforaphane: Abundant in broccoli, cauliflower, brussels sprouts, kale, and green onions, this phytochemical aids the work of enzymes in the body that prevent carcinogens (cancer-causing agents) from damaging healthy cells. Recent studies show that sulforaphane can kill *H. pylori*, the bacteria that causes stomach ulcers—even strains that are resistant to conventional antibiotics.

Try New Foods

Let me clear up a common misconception about healthy eating: Eating a healthy diet doesn't mean you're condemned to eat a boring diet. In fact, despite the proliferation of food choices, most people stick to the same 15 foods and eat them over and over again. (These are not necessarily the 15 *best* foods for you.) Following a limited diet is not only boring, it's also not very satisfying, and I have a hunch it may lead to overeating. In addition, if you are not eating a varied diet, you may be missing out on important vitamins, minerals, and beneficial phytochemicals that can keep your body working at optimal levels and can protect against disease.

For example, if you've never eaten tofu or bean curd, you are denying yourself unique compounds that may protect against certain cancers and even relieve the symptoms of menopause. If you don't know how to prepare tofu, I've included an easy tofu recipe in this book (see page 300). If your fruit intake is restricted to apples and oranges, you are missing out on the spectacular health benefits offered by berries—not just blueberries, but blackberries and raspberries, too. Asian mushrooms, such as shiitake and maitake (trust me, you've eaten them in Japanese and Chinese restaurants), contain powerful anticancer compounds. Once rare in the United States, many big supermarket chains and health-food stores now carry Asian mushrooms in the produce section. They add great flavor and texture to stir-fried dishes. I encourage you to explore some new foods that you may never have eaten before.

CHAPTER 8

THE CURVES MEAL PLAN

Planning for Success

Whether you are following the Carbohydrate-Sensitive Meal Plan or the Calorie-Sensitive Meal Plan, in this chapter I provide all the information that you need to get off to a terrific start.

Your success depends on your ability to find the right food when and where you need it. I show you how to make the best food choices, how to prepare food in a healthy manner, and how to adapt your meal plan so that you can eat at home or eat out without sacrificing your weight-loss goals.

CURVES TIP · Before you begin the Curves Meal Plan, make a shopping list of the foods that you'll need for an entire week. Take the list to the store with you. That way, you'll be sure that your pantry and refrigerator are well stocked with the right food. If you follow my suggested menus, you can use the weekly shopping lists in your Daily Meal Planner.

Meat

A CUT ABOVE · On the food lists in Chapter 4, I have listed the *leanest* cuts of beef, lamb, veal, and pork. All meat is not created equal. Prime beef is not only more expensive than USDA Choice meats, it's also higher in fat content. While you are on Phase 1 and Phase 2, I recommend using Choice meats. In addition, there is a huge difference in calories and fat content among different meats, depending on the cut you choose. For example, a 3.5-ounce serving of short ribs has 285 calories and 18 grams of fat. A similar portion of eye of round roast has 175 calories and 5.7 grams of fat, and a slice of beef tenderloin has 212 calories and 10 grams of fat. Trim as much exterior fat off your meat as you can before cooking it—it is more harmful to you than the fat inside the muscle.

Avoid fatty cuts of pork, such as spare ribs (which can add 21 grams of fat per 3.5-ounce serving!). Loin roast and chops are better alternatives, with about one-third the fat content. Canadian bacon has half the fat content and calories of regular bacon, so it's a better choice.

Cured meats (bacon, hot dogs, and luncheon meats) contain chemicals called "nitrates," which are converted in the stomach into potential cancer-causing agents called "nitrosamines." I know that these are popular foods, but try to use them sparingly or buy the no-nitrate variety sold at some health-food stores and natural-foods supermarkets.

Try some of the newer game meats showing up on menus and in supermarket counters across the country. Buffalo burgers are extremely low in fat and quite delicious, particularly barbequed. Check out the recipe for Buffalo Meatballs on page 292. Venison is also low in fat and calories, and a great alternative to red meat, but if you use venison, be sure that it is tested and free from chronic wasting disease (CWD), an infection similar to mad cow disease that can affect these animals. (There has been no known transmission of CWD from venison to humans, but better to err on the safe side.) At 4 grams of fat and 145 calories per 4-ounce serving, venison is leaner than even the leanest cuts of beef.

NATURAL OR NOT · Many supermarkets and health-food stores sell natural beef that has been raised without growth hormones, antibiotics, or other chemicals. Although these products are not necessary to lose weight, they may offer other health benefits. If they are accessible and affordable, I see no reason not to try them.

COOKING TIPS · Meat can be broiled, grilled, roasted, baked, or sauteed (saute in 1 tablespoon of olive oil or a nonstick spray in a saute pan). Rubs (dry spices) and marinades can help add flavor without extra calories. Hamburgers must be thoroughly cooked to kill disease-causing bacteria, such as E. coli. Do not eat rare hamburgers! The juices should be brown, not red. Beef should be cooked to 160 degrees Fahrenheit, and lamb, veal, and pork should be cooked to 170 degrees.

Poultry

LEAN CHOICE · Chicken, turkey, and Cornish hen are much leaner and have far fewer calories and fat content than red meat. There's one exception, capon, which contains considerably more fat and should be avoided during Phase 1 of the diet. The light meat is lower in calories and fat than the dark meat. While you are on Phase 1 and Phase 2 of the diet, don't eat the turkey or chicken skin, which is where much of the fat collects. Half a roasted chicken breast is 193 calories and about 7.5 grams of fat with the skin and 142 calories and 3.1 grams of fat without the skin. A 3.5-ounce serving of light-meat turkey with the skin is 208 calories and 8.3 grams of fat and without the skin is 157 calories and 3.2 grams of fat. You won't miss the skin, and you certainly won't miss the calories. Ground turkey makes a great burger and is substantially lower in fat and calories than the beef variety.

HANDLE WITH CARE · Raw chicken is often tainted with salmonella, a dangerous bacteria that can cause food poisoning. Cooking the bird thoroughly will kill the bacteria. (If you are roasting chicken, be sure to cook it to 185 degrees.) Never eat rare or red chicken; the juices should be clear. Be especially careful about handling raw chicken in your kitchen or you could inadvertently spread infection. Use a separate cutting board for chicken, and anything that comes in contact with the chicken needs to be thoroughly washed—including your hands.

THE FREE-RANGE OPTION · Unlike most commercially raised chickens and turkeys, free-range poultry are not raised in coops or given antibiotics or hormones to stimulate growth. Free-range poultry is more expensive, but it's worth it if you are worried about ingesting unnecessary chemicals. Calorie counters take note: Free-range birds are often leaner than conventionally raised birds (because they are not as sedentary).

COOKING TIPS · Poultry can be roasted, baked, sauteed, and grilled. Notice that I did not say fried—fried chicken is loaded with calories, extra fat, and trans-fatty acids, and should not be eaten during Phase 1 or Phase 2. If you roast a whole chicken with the skin and peel away the skin after cooking, it may have a bit more flavor and retain more moisture than if you cooked it skinless. Cooking can dry out boneless, skinless chicken breasts and turkey cutlets, so it's best to marinate them for at least two hours before cooking.

CURVES TIP · To save time, marinate poultry in your favorite low-calorie bottled Italian dressing. Since you pour off most of the marinade before cooking, the meat retains only 20 percent of the calories and carbohydrate content from the marinade.

A whole chicken can be simmered slowly on the stove in a pot with vegetables in broth or water to make a wonderful chicken soup, and the boiled chicken can be used to make chicken salad (with low-calorie mayonnaise).

Fish and Seafood

LIGHT AND LEAN · If you are a meat-and-potatoes eater, it's time to learn about the vast variety of fish and seafood that are low in calories and packed with healthy nutrients. An 8-ounce serving of fish, such as flounder, halibut, shrimp, or snapper, is less than 300 calories and has only a few grams of fat. If you just substitute a few fish meals for meat meals every week, you will save yourself hundreds of calories. *If you are on the Calorie-Sensitive Plan, fish is your best protein choice, especially during Phase 1.*

FATTY FISH · Some fish (salmon, tuna, mackerel, sardines) are loaded with good omega-3 fatty acids that are heart healthy and can help keep you in a good mood but are more calorie-dense than low-fat fish. Calorie counters: Remember that fatty fish contains more calories than lean fish, and you should adjust your portion size accordingly. Small, individual cans of tuna or salmon are great for a quick meal with a salad as long as you don't douse them in mayonnaise. Try lemon juice and dijon mustard instead. (If you are counting calories, buy fish that is packed in water, not oil.)

BUYING FISH · Whether you buy fish in a supermarket or fish market, be sure that it is very fresh. Fresh fish does not have a strong fishy smell—it should have a mild odor. If you buy the whole fish, the eyes should be bright and clear. Cloudy eyes mean that fish has been lying around for a while. Fresh fish should be kept for only 24 hours in your refrigerator. Cooked fish can last for about two days. If you don't have access to fresh fish, fresh frozen fish is an excellent alternative. Be sure to buy fish without any added sauces, and follow the instructions on the label to defrost it safely.

COOKING TIPS · Fish can be sauteed, baked, grilled, or poached. Fish is fully cooked when it becomes opaque and flakes easily. Frying fish defeats the purpose of eating fish! It adds lots of bad fat and calories.

PREGNANT WOMEN · Due to environmental pollution, some fish have high levels of methyl mercury that may harm fetal development. The Food and Drug Administration advises pregnant women to eat no more than 12 cooked ounces or about two servings of any type of fish per week and to avoid swordfish, shark, king mackerel, and tilefish. Although it did not ban tuna, the FDA recommends that pregnant women not eat more than two 6-ounce cans of tuna per week. Many physicians, however, feel that pregnant women should steer clear of tuna altogether, given its high mercury content.

Dairy and Eggs

Stick to low-fat or no-fat dairy products most of the time. Cottage cheese, yogurt, and milk are good sources of protein and calcium, a mineral women need for strong bones. Eat only plain yogurt—not fruit-flavored yogurt, which is high in sugar. If you crave fruit, add a bit of fresh fruit to your plain yogurt (but deduct it from your carbohydrate total for the day). You get the benefit of fiber and phytochemicals without all the added sugar.

Cheese is a reasonably good source of both protein and calcium, and as you will see from the menus, I allow some on both meal plans, but in limited quantities because the calories can add up quickly. The good thing is, even a small portion of cheese can be very satisfying.

Eggs fell out of favor, starting in the 1980s, during the cholesterol hysteria. (One egg contains 300 milligrams of cholesterol and about 5 grams of saturated fat.) Recent studies show, however, that eggs do not raise cholesterol in most people, and unless you have high cholesterol and are advised by your doctor not to eat eggs, eating up to two eggs a day seems to be fine. A hard-boiled egg makes a great portable snack, and an omelette is a terrific, high-protein way to start the day. Use a nonstick cooking pan and as little butter or olive oil as possible. Interestingly, scientists now acknowledge that eating cholesterol does not appear to raise cholesterol levels, and that elevated cholesterol is due to other factors.

Fruits and Vegetables

FRESH IS BEST · Fresh produce is your best option, but frozen is a good alternative as long as you don't buy products that are doused in butter, syrup, or other fattening sauces. Canned products not only don't taste as good but often lose vitamins and minerals during processing and may be loaded with added sugar or salt. Sun-ripened, fresh-looking undamaged produce is the best. If available, vine-ripened produce is tastier and more nutrient-dense than the produce allowed to ripen off the vine. You may have to pay a bit more for it, but it's worth it in terms of added flavor.

STORAGE · Fresh fruits and vegetables should be stored in a cool, dry place away from heat and direct sunlight. Ripe fruit (with the exception of bananas) should be refrigerated or it will turn bad. When they are in season (and reasonably priced), fresh berries can be put in a plastic bag and stored in the freezer.

BUYING FROZEN PRODUCE · If you use frozen vegetables or fruits, be sure that the vegetables or fruits are not clumped together in a solid block. That's a sign that the produce has been defrosted and refrozen, which will destroy a significant amount of nutrients. You should be able to feel the individual stalks of broccoli or berries through the package. If it feels like a solid rock, don't buy it.

WASH IT WELL · Most of the phytonutrients are concentrated in the skins of fruits and vegetables. Many people are reluctant to eat the skins, however, due to the use of pesticides used in farming and waxes used on the outside of fruits and vegetables to make them look more attractive and extend shelf life. Washing your produce well in cold water with a scrub brush *used for produce only* and a citrus vegetable wash (sold in most supermarkets) can eliminate much of the chemical residue. I know it's annoying to have to wash your produce every time you grab an apple or make a salad. Many people find it more convenient to wash a few days' worth of produce ahead of time.

Washed lettuce (and other greens) will stay crisp for two to three days in the refrigerator if you wrap a few leaves at a time in paper towels and store them in a plastic bag or in the refrigerator crisper. If you are in a hurry, you can use the prewashed cut-up salads sold in plastic bags in the supermarket produce section. Keep in mind, however, that cut-up, prepackaged salads may have lost some of their nutrients in the processing and handling. Still, it's better than not eating salad at all. Prepared produce from salad bars is fine, as long as the store is clean and the produce is fresh.

Washed, cut-up vegetables (peppers, broccoli, cauliflower) can last for two days, but beyond that they can lose their crispness. Wash your vegetables ahead of time and cut them up as needed. Store them in the refrigerator crisper. *Many vegetables are Free Foods. Keep a supply of ready-to-eat Free Foods in your refrigerator.*

COOKING TIPS · Many vegetables can and should be eaten raw to get the full complement of nutrients. If you like them better cooked, the following are some easy ways to prepare vegetables.

STEAMING IS BEST: If you cook vegetables, do so in as little water as possible, to conserve vitamins and minerals. To steam your vegetables, cut them into small, bite-size pieces and place them in a steamer basket, which you can buy at most supermarkets and houseware and hardware stores. Put a small amount of water in a pot (just enough to reach the steamer basket but not touch the vegetables). Cook over a low flame for three to four minutes after the water is boiling, or until the vegetables are cooked but still crisp. Although most vegetables cook quickly, some tougher vegetables take longer. For example, brussels sprouts can take about 10 minutes to cook, and it can take a full hour to steam an artichoke.

SAUTE: Vegetables can also be sauteed in a nonstick pan with a tablespoon of olive oil or some vegetable or chicken broth, or stir-fried in a small amount of olive oil.

MICROWAVE: Vegetables can also be cooked quickly in a microwave oven in a small amount of water. Keep in mind that microwave cooking can destroy some B vitamins, particularly folic acid. If you use the microwave to cook your vegetables, be sure to take a B-vitamin supplement. Be sure to use microwave-safe dishes! Since microwave ovens vary, check your microwave oven handbook to get the correct cooking time for vegetables.

GRILLED: Some vegetables are great grilled (mushrooms, peppers, and zucchini) and can turn hardcore vegetable haters into vegetable lovers. Cut the vegetables into bite-size pieces, brush them with a little olive oil, season them with a little lemon pepper, and cook them on an outdoor or indoor grill until they are tender. You can even grill them on top of the stove in a grill pan.

ORGANIC OPTION · Organic products are those that are grown or processed without pesticides or other chemical additives. Organic products include fruits and vegetables, as well as products made with organic fruits and vegetables, including grains. At one time it was hard to find organic produce, but today most major supermarkets and health-food stores sell it. Recently, the Department of Agriculture has begun certifying organic products. Those that meet the grade can carry the USDA seal, similar to the seal you see on meat and eggs. There are three types of organic labels. Products that are entirely organic will have a "100 percent organic" label. Products that contain at least 95 percent organic ingredients will have a USDA organic stamp. Products that have at least 70 percent organic ingredients will not have a USDA seal, but can be labeled "made with organic ingredients."

Due to the increased cost of growing and manufacturing, you may pay up to 50 percent more for organic foods than nonorganic. If you can afford it and it's accessible, buying organic is a good way to support farmers and food manufacturers who are trying to do the right thing. If it's a financial hardship for you, however, don't bother. You don't need to use these products to succeed on my program.

CAUTION · Just because produce is labeled organic doesn't mean that it doesn't need to be washed! Organic produce may be prone to fungal or bacterial infection and should be carefully washed, just like other produce.

Breads, Grains, and Pastas

THE REAL THING · The three words to remember are whole, un-processed, and unrefined. If you eliminate bleached white flour, sugar, and processed foods from your daily diet, you will be slimmer and healthier. That means buying whole-grain bread and crackers (with as high a fiber count as possible), brown rice, and whole-wheat pasta. After switching to whole grains, you will wonder how you ever ate the other stuff before!

BAD CHOICES · Bagels, muffins, croissants, pancakes, and waffles are loaded with carbohydrates, and we tend to make them even worse by pouring on added fat and sugar such as butter, cream cheese, syrup, or jams. If you start your day with these foods, by mid-morning you will be ravenous and craving more.

BEST CEREALS · Look for cereals with a high fiber and high protein content. I've seen some brands that contain as much as 9 grams of protein and 10 grams of fiber per 1-cup serving. If you want to turn a low-protein cereal into a high-protein cereal, you can add a scoop or two of protein powder to a bowl of warm oatmeal or Wheatena.

CARB ADDICTS BEWARE · Keep in mind that even good grains are high in carbohydrates and can be a problem for carbohydrate-sensitive people. The fact is, the more grains you eat, the less fat you will burn. If you want to stay in fat-burning mode, limit your portions.

Seeds and Nuts

JUST A TASTE · Seeds and nuts are high in calories and fat (albeit the good monounsaturated fat), so use them sparingly. I include them in Phases 1 and 2 of the meal plans for three reasons: (1) People love them. (2) Numerous studies have documented that people who eat nuts are less likely to get heart disease. (3) They add pizzazz to bland foods like cottage cheese. Those are good enough reasons for me. The key is to watch your portion size. One ounce (a small handful) of almonds has 166 calories, 15 grams of fat, and only 1.4 grams of protein. The same amount of cashews contains 163 calories, 13 grams of fat, and 4.35 grams of protein. Peanuts, which are actually a legume, or bean, but are eaten like nuts, have more protein at 7 grams per ounce, but roughly the same amount of calories and fat. Remember, a 1-ounce portion is very little, and most people can down a few handfuls of nuts in a matter of minutes. If you need to eat something crunchy and are counting calories, pumpkin seeds are a better choice. They are 110 calories per ounce, with 5 grams of protein and 5 grams of fat.

NUT BUTTERS · Nut butters contain a bit more protein than nuts, but they are high in fat, and you have to be vigilant about portion size. Two tablespoons of peanut butter is about 190 calories and close to 8 grams of protein. If you can limit your portion size to 2 tablespoons, it's fine, but if you need to eat half a container to feel satisfied, it's not the best choice for you, especially if you're counting calories. Almond butter and cashew butter are sold in health-food stores, and they're quite delicious, but once again, a little goes a long way.

BEWARE OF TRAIL MIX · Commercially prepared trail mix is usually a blend of nuts, seeds, and dried fruits. The dried fruits are loaded with sugar and calories. You can save hundreds of calories and dozens of carb grams by making your own seed-and-nut mix minus the dried fruit.

Legumes

HIDDEN CARBOHYDRATES · Legumes include lentils, kidney beans, soybeans, black beans, and garbanzo beans. Although legumes contain a fair amount of protein, they are also loaded with carbohydrates. For example, ½ cup of cooked lentils is 8 grams of protein and nearly 20 grams of carbohydrates. The exception is tofu, a bean curd made from soybeans, which is low in carbohydrates—less than 1 gram of carbohydrates and 10 grams of protein per ½-cup serving. Soy is the only legume that is a complete protein, which means you can substitute it for meat. (Most legumes are incomplete proteins and must be eaten with grains to form a complete protein.)

GREAT SOURCE OF FIBER · Legumes are a great source of fiber, so at least some of the carbohydrates in them are indigestible. If you want to increase your fiber intake, you can add cooked kidney beans or garbanzo beans to your salads (you'll see them in many salad bars) or eat them as a side dish. Remember, however, that ½ cup of beans can easily add 100 calories to your salad or meal.

Condiments

The wrong condiments can add a surprising amount of calories and carbohydrates to your meals. Read labels! There is a tremendous disparity among brands. For example, some brands of ketchup have up to 7 grams of carbohydrates per serving, while others have between 2 and 4. Steak sauce can also be loaded with sugar. We often recommend that people use a small amount of barbeque sauce instead of ketchup or steak sauce because many brands contain less carbohydrates.

Mayonnaise is usually pure fat, so it doesn't contain any carbohydrates, but it can be calorie dense. If you are on the Calorie-Sensitive Meal Plan, you may be better off using low-calorie mayonnaise, which usually has about half the calories of regular mayonnaise, although it contains 1 gram of carbohydrate.

Use as much yellow mustard and lemon juice as you like as seasonings. These condiments are Free Foods. (See page 58.)

If you do not have to watch your sodium intake, you can use soy sauce, which usually does not contain any carbohydrates, but teriyaki sauce has lots of added sugar, which adds up to more carbohydrates.

Horseradish is a great option for sandwiches. It's made from radishes (which is another Free Food) and adds lots of flavor with no carbohydrates and minimal calories.

Commercial salad dressings can be tricky. Beware of no-fat salad dressings: They can be loaded with sugar and high in carbohydrates.

Low-calorie salad dressings are often a better choice, as long as they do not contain more than 50 calories and 4 grams of carbohydrate per 2-tablespoon serving. My personal preference is a small amount of olive oil with lemon juice or vinegar.

Keeping Track

WHAT'S A PORTION? · Since few of us walk around with food scales or rulers, you need to be able to size up your food quickly. Here are some easy ways to keep track of your portion sizes.

MEAT, FISH, AND POULTRY: A 4-ounce serving of meat, fish, or poultry is slightly bigger than the size of a deck of cards or the palm of a woman's hand. You will eat between 4 and 6 ounces of protein per meal.

DAIRY: ½ cup of cottage cheese or plain yogurt is about the size of a tennis ball. 1 ounce of hard cheese is about the size of a third of your fist or 4 stacked dice. 1 piece of presliced cheese is about 1 ounce.

VEGETABLES: 1 cup of broccoli is about the size of your fist (from the wrist to the tip of the knuckles).

FRUIT: 1 medium-size apple or peach is about the size of a tennis ball. ½ cup of berries or sliced fruit is half the size of your fist.

GRAINS AND CEREALS: 1 cup of cooked pasta, cooked rice, or cereal is about the size of your fist.

NUTS: 1 ounce of seeds or nuts is one moderately filled (not stuffed) handful.

BUTTER: 1 teaspoon of butter or peanut butter is about the size of your thumb from the top of the knuckle to the fingertip.

How to Read a Food Label

The Food Lists in Chapter 4 have provided information on the calorie and carbohydrate content of commonly consumed foods that I consider to be optimal for the Curves Meal Plan. Please try to build your menus around these foods. For the sake of variety, I have added additional foods in my sample menus, but in limited quantities.

- Those of you following the Carbohydrate-Sensitive Plan will keep track of your daily carbohydrate intake.
- Those following the Calorie-Sensitive Plan will keep track of your daily carbohydrate and calorie intake.

Given the variety of foods in today's supermarkets, however, it's impossible for me to list everything here. I recommend that you purchase one of the many food guides on the market that list the nutrient values of common foods, including the carbohydrate and calorie content. Corrine T. Netzer's *Complete Book of Food Counts* (Dell, 2000) is an excellent choice and is worth the $7.95 investment. This guide lists many of the brand-name products that you probably use in your home. However, manufacturers can change a product's ingredients overnight, so you can't always count on a food guide. Fortunately, many foods come packaged with nutritional labels that will help you keep track of what you are eating. See the sample food label on page 161. Here are some tips on how to read food labels.

SERVING SIZE: The information on food labels reflects *one* serving size. Serving size is supposed to be standardized to reflect the typical portion normally eaten by the average person so that consumers can compare the nutrient value of similar products. Despite the government's attempt to standardize portions, similar products are not always labeled the same way. For example, the serving size for some brands of bread is one slice, and for others the serving size is two or even three slices. Some brands of cereal use 1 cup as a serving size, others use ¾ cup or even ½ cup. When you are tracking calories and carbohydrates, read the label carefully so you can write down the correct total.

Nutrition Facts
Serving Size 1 cup (34g)
Servings Per Container about 10

Amount Per Serving	Cereal	Cereal with 1/2 cup skim milk
Calories	110	150
Calories from Fat	15	15

	% Daily Value**	
Total Fat 1.5g*	2%	3%
Saturated Fat 0g	0%	0%
Polyunsaturated Fat 1g		
Monounsaturated Fat 0.5g		
Cholesterol 0mg	0%	0%
Sodium 0mg	0%	3%
Potassium 90mg	3%	8%
Total Carbohydrate 22g	7%	9%
Dietary Fiber 2g	8%	8%
Sugars 3g		
Protein 4g		
Vitamin A	0%	6%
Vitamin C	30%	35%
Calcium	0%	15%
Iron	10%	10%
Thiamin	8%	10%
Riboflavin	0%	10%
Niacin	2%	4%

*Amount in cereal. One half cup skim milk contributes an additional 40 calories, 65mg sodium, 6g total carbohydrate (6g sugars), and 4g protein.
**Percent Daily Values are based on a 2,000 calorie diet. Your daily values may be higher or lower depending on your calorie needs:

	Calories:	2,000	2,500
Total Fat	Less than	65g	80g
Sat Fat	Less than	20g	25g
Cholesterol	Less than	300mg	300mg
Sodium	Less than	2,400mg	2,400mg
Total Carbohydrate		300g	375g
Dietary Fiber		25g	30g

Sample Food Label

CALORIES: Calories are listed per serving size.

CALORIES FROM FAT: the percentage of calories from all forms of fat

% DAILY VALUE: This figure shows how each food fits into a normal 2,000-calorie diet. This is a guideline to help people make better food choices. For example, if a food derives 50 percent of its calories from fat, and the goal is to eat a diet with 30 percent of its calories from fat, that's a red flag that this food is too high in fat and that you need to limit your consumption of this food.

TOTAL FAT*: This is the total number of all fat grams in a product.

SATURATED FAT: amount of saturated fat grams per serving

CHOLESTEROL: total number of cholesterol grams per serving

SODIUM: total sodium content per serving

TOTAL CARBOHYDRATES: total grams of carbohydrates per serving

DIETARY FIBER: total grams of fiber per serving

SUGARS: includes naturally occurring sugars as well as added sugars

PROTEIN: total grams of protein per serving

VITAMINS AND MINERALS: These figures are based on the U.S. Dietary Reference Intakes. Only vitamins A and C, calcium, and iron are required to be included on the food label. A manufacturer can voluntarily list other vitamins, minerals, and phytochemicals.

Tips for Eating Out

For someone trying to lose weight, eating out is a double-edged sword. The upside: You can't beat the convenience, and when someone else prepares your meals, you're not hanging around the kitchen tempted by food. The downside: You're exposed to a whole menu filled with food that could get you into trouble, not to mention the bread on the table and the dessert tray.

*What's missing—There is no value for polyunsaturated fat or trans-fatty acids, which can be just as harmful, if not more so, than saturated fat.

On the Curves Meal Plan, you don't have to forgo the convenience of eating out to succeed. With some planning ahead of time, you can eat out without blowing Phase 1 or Phase 2.

SELECT A HEALTH-CONSCIOUS RESTAURANT • When you choose the restaurant, be sure that there is something on the menu that you can eat. A pizzeria is a bad choice if you are on the Calorie-Sensitive or Carbohydrate-Sensitive Plans, but an Italian restaurant that offers salads and meat or fish entrees is workable. Diners are great because they typically have a wide variety of food and serve it without a lot of fancy sauces. Asian restaurants are a great option as long as you order the steamed or lightly sauteed vegetables with fish or chicken and avoid the deep-fried selections or food cooked in heavy sauces. Fast-food restaurants are okay as long as you order a burger or grilled chicken sandwich (throw away the bun) and a side salad. If you are counting calories, do not "super size" your order—the Quarter Pounder is the perfect portion size for you. And of course, don't order the fries. Even an all-you-can-eat buffet is fine if you're committed to sticking with the lean protein entrees with vegetables and salads. Fill your plate with Free Foods (isn't it nice to have someone else prepare the vegetables for a change?), and bypass the starches and desserts. Just make sure that the vegetables are not cooked in butter. If you find that you can't resist temptation, buffets are not the restaurants for you.

PLAN AHEAD • Before you pick up the menu, have an idea of what you're going to order. Look for a lean protein option (such as grilled or broiled chicken, small fish fillet, or a turkey burger) with steamed vegetables on the side and a salad. Take advantage of your Free Foods. They will fill you up fast.

GIVE CAREFUL INSTRUCTIONS • Let your server know that you want your food cooked "clean," without butter or sauces. Ask for any dressing or gravy to be served on the side, and use it sparingly, if at all. A tablespoon of olive oil with lemon juice or vinegar makes a great salad dressing and is lower in calories than most commercial dressings.

WATCH YOUR PORTION SIZES · If you are counting calories, please note that many restaurants serve huge meat, poultry, and fish portions. Share the entree with someone else, or cut off the right amount for your meal and ask for a doggie bag to bring the rest of the food home. You can use it for another meal.

Eating on the Job Should Not Be a Chore

The Curves Meal Plan is easy to follow if you work outside the home, as long as you plan ahead. Since you will be eating several of your six meals away from home, you will need to bring the appropriate food with you every day. Here are some tips on how to make it easy to stay on your diet at work.

- Carry a container of Free Foods with you at all times.
- Take a Curves Shake or other protein shake to work with you every day. It counts as a meal.
- Keep individual cans of tuna, salmon, or canned chicken in your desk or locker for a quick meal with your cut-up vegetables.
- If you have access to a refrigerator at work, stock it at the beginning of the week with low-fat cottage cheese, yogurt, prepackaged salad, and other foods that will help you put together a quick meal.
- If you bring salad to work, pack the lettuce in one container and the wet ingredients (tomato, cucumber) in another, and mix them together when you are ready for your meal. Top your salad with some leftover chicken breast or lean, sliced steak, add a small amount of low-carbohydrate dressing, and you have a perfect meal.
- Cook an extra portion of chicken, meat, or fish the night before so you have it for lunch the next day. Store it overnight in the same container that you will bring to work.

CHAPTER 9

THE CURVES AT-HOME WORKOUT

recently received an interesting phone call from a friend who works out with a personal trainer at her gym. She told me that she had complained to her trainer that the workouts were becoming too time-consuming and that she just wasn't getting enough out of them.

Her trainer responded, "I have a great idea. Why don't we do a Curves-style workout?"

When I heard that story, I realized that we had achieved our mission—the Curves-style workout had become a new exercise model for women.

What is a Curves-style workout, and what makes it so unique? The Curves Workout incorporates the three major components of fitness—strength training, cardiovascular training, and stretching—in a simple 30-minute routine that you do three times a week. It's a truly efficient workout—you don't waste a minute—yet it is highly effective. By the time the half-hour is over, you will:

1. strengthen every major muscle group,
2. give your heart and lungs a good aerobic workout,
3. increase the flexibility of your joints, and
4. feel energized and ready to get back to your busy day.

Millions of women have benefited from the Curves Workout at Curves, and now you can do a Curves-style workout at home. It's fast, effective, and fun. And the best part is, you don't need a lot of fancy equipment. The only thing you need to buy is an exercise resistance tube—a thin rubber tube that takes the place of weights and machines. Be sure to get an exercise *tube,* not an exercise *band.* An exercise tube is more like a rubber rope, and an exercise band is wider. Be sure to buy an exercise tube that comes with two handles, one on each end. Make sure that the tube has *soft, flexible* handles that can bend. Some exercises require that you put your foot through the handle. Exercise tubes can be purchased in different lengths. The Curves At-Home Workout is designed for a four-foot-long tube, which can cost anywhere from $5.99 to $30, depending on the brand and how many tubes are included in the set. You can buy your exercise tube at a sporting-goods store, a discount general-merchandise store such as Wal-Mart, or even on the Internet. *Be sure to buy a tube that is four feet long—the exercises will not work on a tube that is too short or too long.*

You don't need to buy any fancy exercise clothing unless you want to, but do wear comfortable, nonbinding clothes. Shorts, yoga pants, or sweatpants are fine. A sturdy pair of athletic shoes with ridges on the bottom is a *must.* There are times when you will wrap the tube around your shoes, and if the surface is too slippery, the tube will not stay in place.

You can do the Curves At-Home Workout anywhere in your home, as long as you have access to a sturdy, straight-back chair and a doorknob that will not pull off if you yank it too hard.

The Three Components of Fitness

STRENGTH TRAINING   There's only one way to protect and make new muscle: You have to make your muscles work harder than they are used to working. The same rules apply whether you are pumping iron or using an exercise tube.

- If you are working with an exercise tube, the tension on the tube must be strong enough to resist the pull of your muscles. (That's why weight training is also called *resistance* training.)
- If you are working on a standard exercise machine, choose a weight that is sufficiently challenging so that your muscles are fatigued after the first set.

CURVES TIP   Working against resistance that is too light or too easy does not make muscle. In recent years, it's become popular to hand out 1-pound weights in aerobics classes and tell women that they are strength training while they are doing aerobics. Holding low weights during an aerobic workout will merely enhance the intensity of the aerobic workout and will have no effect on muscle.

CARDIOVASCULAR TRAINING   "Cardio" (also called aerobic exercise) is any exercise that elevates your heart to your target or training level and sustains it for 20 minutes or more. Your heart is a muscle, and it also needs to work harder than it normally does to get stronger, but you don't want to overwork it. You should work at a pace that is challenging but not exhausting. Cardiovascular exercise strengthens your heart and lungs, and helps your muscles better utilize energy and rid themselves of waste products. It also promotes fat burning. (Please read "Working Safely: Finding Your Targetr Heart Rate or Training Level" on page 168.)

STRETCHING   As people age, their joints become stiffer and their bodies less flexible. Stretching helps to maintain more fluid joints (which means less pain and better range of motion), enhances the effectiveness of resistance training, improves balance, and reduces the risk of back injury. It also feels great and should be done at the end of every workout. (See the Curves Flexibility Exercises on pages 186–87.)

Working Safely: Finding Your Target Heart Rate or Training Level

Use this simple formula to determine your target heart rate or training level.

(1) Subtract your age from 220 (that gives you your maximum heart rate—you never want to exceed this rate because it could put too much strain on your heart).

(2) Multiply that number by 50 to 80 percent to get your target heart rate. Someone in good health should work at about 65 percent of her target heart rate. For example, here is how a 50-year-old woman in good health would determine her target heart rate:

220 − 50 = 170, or your maximum heart rate

170 × .65 = 110

That means that while you are working out, your heart should beat 110 times per minute. How can you tell how fast your heart is beating? You can measure your heart rate by feeling your pulse on your wrist or on your carotid artery on your neck. If your heart is beating 110 times per minute, every 10 seconds it should beat about 18 times. If your heart rate is above the target, work at a slower pace. If it's below the target, increase the intensity of your workout.

Don't like math? On page 169, you will find a simple chart that will help you determine how to measure your target heart rate based on your age.

CURVES TIP · If you are just beginning an exercise regimen, or if you have a health problem such as diabetes, high blood pressure, or heart disease, you should work at the lower level (50 percent). Therefore, if you are 50 years old, you would determine your training heart rate by subtracting 50 from 220, and then multiplying that number by 50 percent (or .50). Of course, check with your physician before doing these or any other exercises.

Fitting It All In

How can you accomplish a total-body workout in such a short period of time? The formula is simple—you make every second count. If

TARGET HEART RATE CHART
(10 Second Count)

Curves ™

Find your pulse with either of the two methods. Count the number of times your heart beats during 10 seconds starting with zero. The 50% level of intensity is for special populations with conditions such as pregnancy, hypertension and obesity. Choose the target heart rate level that is appropriate for you. Always err to the side of caution. You should seek the advice of a physician before beginning any exercise program.

Carotid Pulse
To find and count the carotid pulse place the index and middle fingers gently on the side of the neck, next to the throat. Be careful to press down lightly.

Radial Pulse
The radial pulse can be found by placing the first two fingers lightly over the radial artery of the wrist. It is directly in line with the thumb.

AGE	50%	60%	70%	80%	85%
15	17	21	24	27	29
20	17	20	23	27	28
25	16	19	23	26	28
30	16	19	22	25	27
35	15	19	22	25	26
40	15	18	21	24	26
45	15	18	20	23	25
50	14	17	20	23	24
55	14	17	19	22	23
60	13	16	19	21	23
65	13	16	18	21	22
70	13	15	18	20	21
75	12	15	17	19	21
80	12	14	16	19	20

you've ever worked out at a gym, you know that the standard workout requires a minimum of an hour and a half. With other programs, you do a five-minute warm-up, usually on a cardio machine. Before you place an added load on your muscles, you want to warm them up—that is, get the blood flowing to your muscles so that they have more oxygen and nutrients to do the extra work. This makes your muscles more elastic and less susceptible to injury.

Then you move on to weight training. That can be a huge time waster! In reality, you spend only *half* your time engaging in actual exercise because you have to rest your muscles between sets. For example, if you're working out on a chest machine, you will typically do 10 to 12 repetitions of an exercise (that's one set) and then have to wait a few minutes before doing the next set of repetitions to allow your muscles time to recover. If you work all of your muscles, it can take up to an hour! After you've done all your weight training, you still need to do 20 minutes of cardio and then a cooldown. (The last few minutes of your workout should be done at a progressively slower pace to allow your body to adjust back to normal.) You still haven't done your stretching, and unfortunately that's the part most people skip! This method of working out is fine for women who aren't trying to squeeze exercise into a tight lunch break or who don't have to pick kids up at school or run home to cook dinner. But it doesn't work for most women who do.

The Curves Workout at home (or at Curves) revolutionizes the standard workout in several key ways. *The magic of the Curves workout is that you do strength training and cardio at the same time, eliminating the wasteful rest between sets and the need to do cardio before or after your strength training.* There's even some time left over at the end for stretching. We have streamlined the standard workout in other key ways. We do shorter exercise intervals, but not at the expense of muscle. The fact is, you don't make stronger muscles by lifting the same weight over and over again. *Short bursts of intense activities are the best way to increase muscle strength.* The first 30 seconds of any exercise is when your muscles work the hardest. After that, it's all downhill, so why do repetition after repetition? In the Curves At-Home Workout, you do as many repetitions as you can in 40 seconds for each exercise (that gives you time to get into your position and make any adjustment to your equipment) and then move on to another using a different muscle group, which gives your muscles plenty of time to rest. When you are done doing one set of all your exercises, you go back and do the second set.

In the Curves At-Home Workout, you don't lose momentum during recovery time, when your muscles are resting. You continue an aerobic-type activity that will maintain your target heart rate—*that's why I call it the Aerobic Recovery.* At Curves, we have Recovery Stations between pieces of exercise equipment. If you are working out at home or in the gym, you create your own Recovery Station. Any activity that keeps you moving in a lively fashion is fine. You can walk rapidly up and down your stairs, or you can step on and off the bottom step, or you can run in place or jump rope (if you don't have knee or joint problems), or you can use an exercise bike (many people have these at home but don't use them!). You can do any activity for 40 seconds that maintains your target heart rate.

After the Aerobic Recovery interlude, you return to your resistance training but work an opposite muscle group. That is, you alternate upper body and lower body exercises. Here's how it works:

1. If you have just done a chest exercise or other upper-body exercise before your Aerobic Recovery, you will now do a leg or lower-body exercise. (Those upper-body muscles still need some time off.)
2. After 40 seconds of exercising, do your Aerobic Recovery for another 40 seconds to give your muscles a rest while at the same time maintaining your target heart rate.
3. After 40 seconds of Aerobic Recovery, do an upper-body exercise for 40 seconds, and so on.

CURVES TIP · When you first embark on the Curves At-Home Workout, allow yourself some extra time to become familiar with the exercises and the routine. After you do it a few times, you will be able to zip right through it.

The Curves At-Home Workout at a Glance

The Three-Minute Warm-Up
1. Straight Crunches
2. Side (Oblique) Crunches

Combination Cardio/Strength Training
3. Chest Press
   Aerobic Recovery
4. Leg Extension
   Aerobic Recovery
5. Back Row
   Aerobic Recovery
6. Leg Curl
   Aerobic Recovery
7. Shoulder Press
   Aerobic Recovery
8. Squat
   Aerobic Recovery
9. Lat Pull
   Aerobic Recovery
10. Back Raise
   Aerobic Recovery

When you have completed one set of Cardio/Strength Training, do a second set.

Cooldown
11. Hip Abductor, right leg
12. Hip Adductor, right leg
   Aerobic Recovery
13. Hip Abductor, left leg
14. Hip Adductor, left leg
   Aerobic Recovery

Stretching
The Curves Flexibility Exercises

Exercises

The Three-Minute Warm-Up

1 • **STRAIGHT CRUNCHES** • The Abdominals

1. Lie down with your back and your feet flat on the floor and your knees up. Place your hands over your head.*
2. Flex your abdominal muscles to lift your head and upper torso into a crunch. Use your hands as a guide only.
3. Exhale as you come up; inhale as you go down.
4. Do as many straight crunches as you can in 90 seconds. Over time, work up to 50 crunches.

*You may need to put your hands behind your head and neck for additional support. Be careful not to pull up against your head or neck, and do not yank your head or neck, as it can cause injury. Let your adominal muscles do all the work.

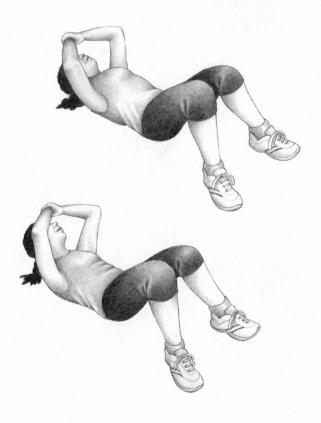

2 · SIDE (OBLIQUE) CRUNCHES · The Obliques

1. In the same position as the straight crunch, flex your abdominal muscles, but this time twist to your left side simultaneously in one smooth movement.
2. Exhale as you go up; inhale as you go down.
3. Flex your abdominal muscles and twist to your right side simultaneously in one smooth movement.
4. Alternate twisting from your right and left sides for about 90 seconds. Work up to 50 oblique crunches.

NO AEROBIC RECOVERY · Move right on to Cardio/Strength Training.

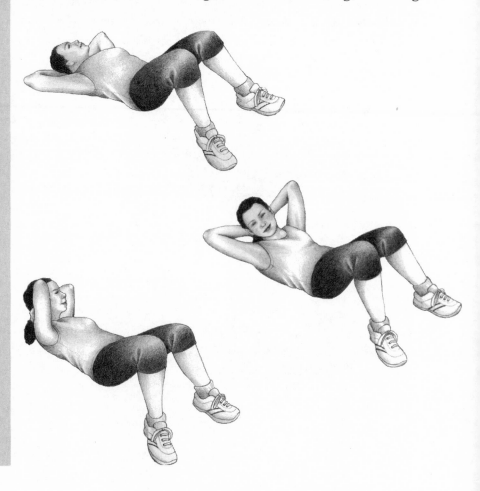

Combination Cardio/Strength Training

Once you have completed the first set of the following exercises, go back and do a second set.

3 • **CHEST PRESS** • Upper Body: Pectorals

1. Place your exercise tube around a doorknob (with the door closed) and stand or sit in a chair with your back to the door.
2. Move far enough away from the door to extend the tube for adequate resistance.
3. Grasp one handle in each hand and push forward from chest height.
4. Push as far as you can, and then return to starting position. *Be sure to move out directly in front of your chest, keeping your elbows aligned with the movement.*
5. Perform as many repetitions as you can in 40 seconds.

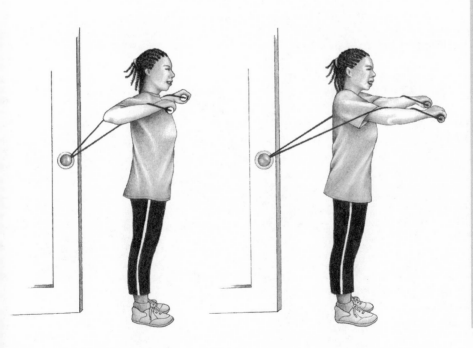

AEROBIC RECOVERY • 40 seconds

> Do any activity that keeps you moving and helps you maintain your target heart rate while giving your muscles time to rest. Try walking quickly up the stairs, running in place, jumping rope, doing jumping jacks, or stepping up and down on a step (either the bottom step on your staircase or a step board). Check your target heart rate. If it's too high, work at a slower pace (do fewer repetitions when you do the next exercise). If it's not high enough, work a bit harder. Don't overdo it! Running and jumping can stress your joints, especially if you are arthritic or overweight.

4 • LEG EXTENSION • Lower Body: Quadriceps

1. Sitting in a chair, place the tube around the bottom of both feet and grip with both hands. (Be sure to wear athletic shoes with grooves on the bottoms.) Your hands should be on the edge of the chair near your knees.
2. Grasp the tube rather than the handles, to obtain adequate resistance.
3. Extend both legs until straight. Return both legs to the bent position.
4. Do as many repetitions as you can in 40 seconds.

AEROBIC RECOVERY • 40 seconds

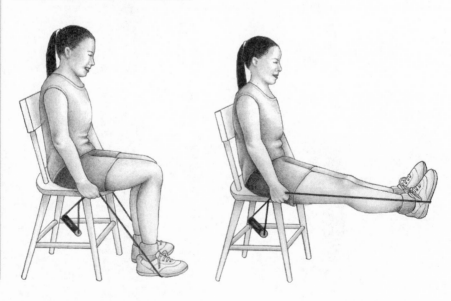

5 • **BACK ROW** • Upper Body: Rhomboids and Latissimus

1. Place the tube around a doorknob (with the door closed) and stand facing the door at an appropriate distance to create adequate resistance.
2. Grasp both handles with arms extended at shoulder height. Stand erect with your knees slightly bent.
3. Pull the handles back to your chest, and keep your elbows aligned at shoulder level.
4. Return to starting position.
5. Do as many repetitions as you can in 40 seconds.

AEROBIC RECOVERY • 40 seconds

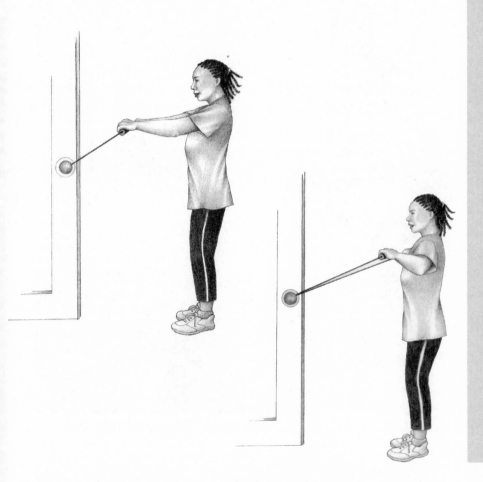

6 · LEG CURL · Lower Body: Hamstrings

1. Stand facing the back of a chair, and hold the chair for stability.
2. Place the tube over the top of the chair and through the bottom. You can create greater resistance by holding the tube rather than the handles, to shorten its length.
3. Place one handle on the bottom of your right or left shoe.
4. With your thigh against the chair back, lift your foot.
5. Perform the first set with one leg, and when you redo this exercise in the second set, use the other leg.
6. Do as many repetitions as you can in 40 seconds.

AEROBIC RECOVERY · 40 seconds

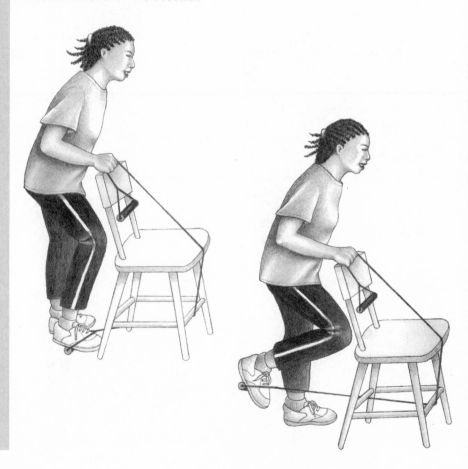

Exercises

7 • **SHOULDER PRESS** • Upper Body: Deltoids

1. Step on the middle of the tube, with handles in each hand. Hands should be at shoulder height with palms facing forward.
2. Press the tube above your head until your arms are almost straight, then lower your arms. Be careful not to straighten the arms completely, to protect the elbow joints.
3. Do as many repetitions as you can in 40 seconds.

AEROBIC RECOVERY • 40 seconds

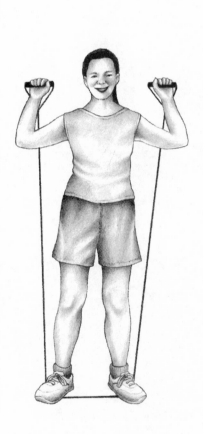
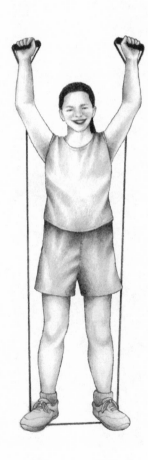

8 • SQUAT • Lower Body: Quadriceps and Gluteus Maximus

1. Stand on the tube with your feet shoulder width apart. Bring the handles up behind your arms and rest them on your shoulders.
2. While keeping your back straight and your stomach tight, slowly squat down until your thighs are parallel to the floor. Be sure to allow your knees to go forward but not past your toes. Arch your back slightly, and extend your behind backward.
3. Raise your body to an upright position.
4. Do as many repetitions as you can in 40 seconds.

AEROBIC RECOVERY • 40 seconds

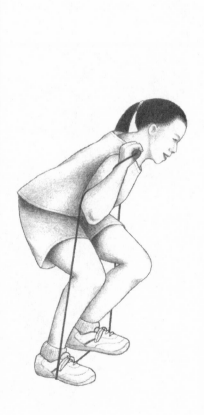
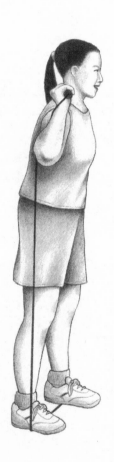

9 • **LAT PULL** • Upper Body: Latissimus

1. Place the tube around a doorknob (with the door closed) and grasp a handle in each hand.
2. Step away the appropriate distance, facing the door, to obtain adequate resistance.
3. Lean forward with arms extended. Keep your head higher than your heart. Pull handles to shoulders.
4. Extend arms, and return to starting position.
5. Do as many repetitions as you can in 40 seconds.

AEROBIC RECOVERY • 40 seconds

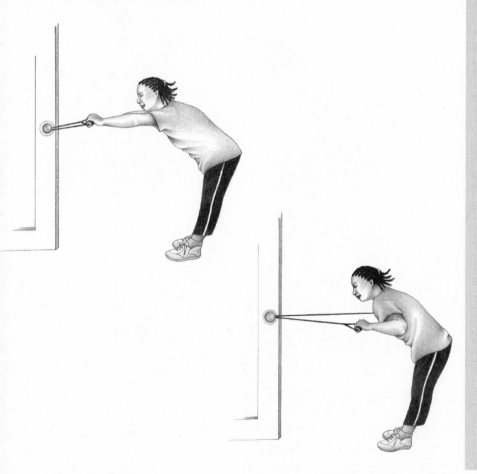

Exercises

10 • BACK RAISE • Upper Body: Spinea Erectors or Lower Back

1. Sit in a chair and place the tube beneath both feet.
2. Lean forward and grasp the tube at the appropriate length to obtain adequate resistance, with hands against the chest.
3. Lift your torso up, and then return to starting position.
4. Do as many repetitions as you can in 40 seconds.

AEROBIC RECOVERY • 40 seconds

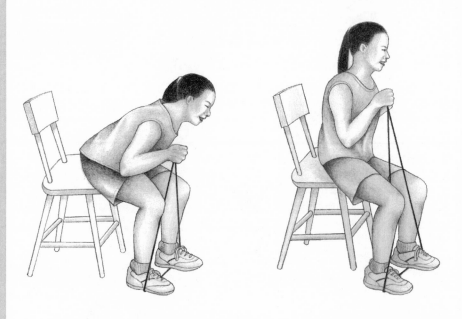

Do another set of each of the resistance-training exercises. When you have completed two sets of the resistance-training exercises, it's time to do your cooldown.

Cooldown

You can continue your exercise routine but allow your heart rate to return to normal by doing these leg exercises, which isolate small muscles and do not require your body to work as hard as it has been working.

11 · HIP ABDUCTOR · Lower Body: Outer Thigh, Right Leg

1. Stand with your left side a few inches from the back of a chair.
2. Place the tube around the chair from the top and through the bottom.
3. Hold one handle with your left hand against the chair back, and place your right foot through the other handle.
4. Extend your right leg away from the chair, and then return to the starting position.
5. Do as many repetitions as you can in 40 seconds.

NO AEROBIC RECOVERY · Stay in position.

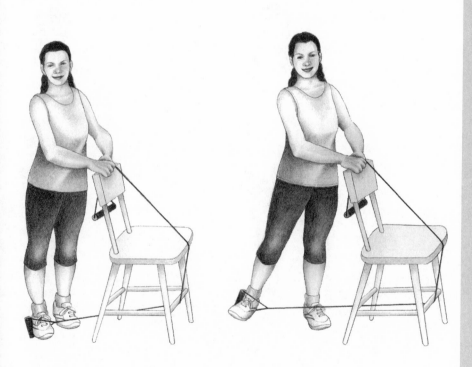

12 · HIP ADDUCTOR · Lower Body: Inner Thigh, Right Leg

1. Now turn and stand with your *right* side toward the chair.
2. Start with your right leg against the chair and legs slightly apart.
3. Extend your right leg away from the chair, across and in front of the left leg.
4. Return to the starting position.
5. Do as many repetitions as you can in 40 seconds.

AEROBIC RECOVERY · 40 seconds

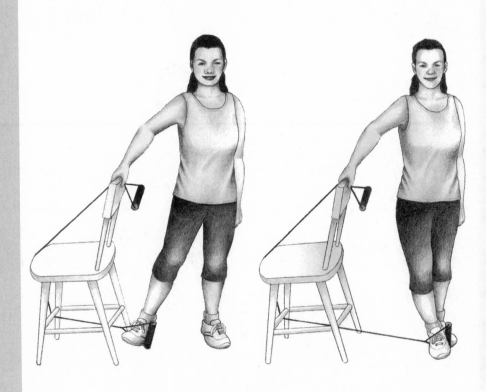

Exercises

13 · HIP ABDUCTOR · Lower Body: Outer Thigh, Left Leg

1. Stand with your right side a few inches from the back of a chair.
2. Place the tube around the chair from the top and through the bottom.
3. Hold one handle with your right hand against the chair back, and place your left foot through the other handle.
4. Extend your left leg away from the chair, and then return to the starting position.
5. Do as many repetitions as you can in 40 seconds.

NO AEROBIC RECOVERY · Stay in position.

14 · HIP ADDUCTOR · Lower Body: Inner Thigh, Left Leg

1. Now turn and stand with your *left* side toward the chair.
2. Start with your left leg against the chair and legs slightly apart.
3. Extend your left leg away from the chair, across and in front of the right leg.
4. Return to the starting position.
5. Do as many repetitions as you can in 40 seconds.

AEROBIC RECOVERY · 40 seconds

Stretching

The final component of a total workout is stretching. The easy-to-follow Curves Flexibility Exercises will show you how to do 12 simple stretches.

1. Hold each stretch for seven seconds and then gently extend further for another seven seconds.
2. Please perform the stretches in the proper order. It's important to do the standing stretches first, before you do the floor stretches. If you place your head below your heart when your heart rate is elevated, you could feel faint. *Remember not to bob, bounce, or force your stretches.*

Curves Flexibility Exercises

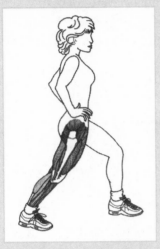

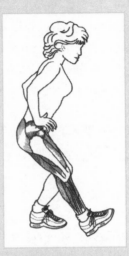

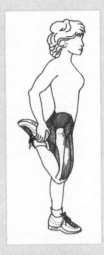

1 • Stand with one leg forward, knee bent, and the other leg behind and straight. Keep heel and foot of the back leg flat against the floor during stretching.

2 • Extend one leg with knee slightly bent and the toe pointing upward. Slowly lower the body, carefully maintaining balance.

3 • Stand on one leg, grasp foot, and gently pull up and back toward the buttocks. Keep pelvis straight and torso upright.

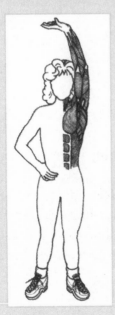

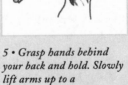

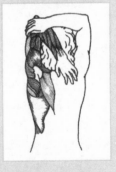

5 • Grasp hands behind your back and hold. Slowly lift arms up to a comfortable tightness.

6 • Grasp your elbow with the opposite hand and gently pull toward your head.

4 • With your feet about shoulder width apart and knees bent, extend one arm overhead and reach down and across the body with the other arm.

Curves Flexibility Exercises

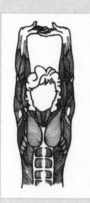

7 • Interlock fingers above your head, push palms upward, and hold after you reach the point of tightness.

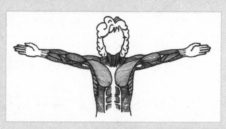

8 • With your arms up and out, palms forward, gently pull the arms back until you feel a tightness in the chest, shoulders, and arm muscles.

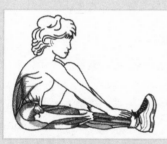

10 • Sit on the floor with one leg bent, your knee to the chest, and the other leg straight. Lean forward, reaching out toward your toes.

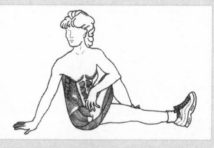

9 • Sit with one leg crossing over and in front of the other leg. Place your elbow on the knee and gently push.

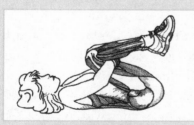

12 • While holding your back flat, grasp your thighs below the knees and pull in toward your chest.

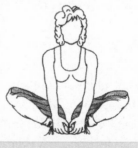

11 • In a sitting position, while holding your feet, place the soles of your shoes together. Let your thighs relax toward the floor. For extra pressure, place your elbows on the inside of your thighs and gently push down.

CHAPTER 10

ENHANCING YOUR
WORKOUT AT CURVES

F ast. Effective. Fun.

These three words best describe the Curves Workout.

FAST: You're in and out in about 30 minutes. That's it. That includes warm-up, strength training, cardio, cooldown, and stretching. There is no adjusting machines, or moving weight stacks, or waiting for machines to become free, or any of the other annoying stuff that eats up your time and does nothing for your body.

EFFECTIVE: The Curves Workout combines cardiovascular training with strength training, which dramatically *increases* the effectiveness of your workout while significantly *reducing* the amount of time you need to spend working out. You also get a lot more bang for your buck out of each exercise. Why? Unlike conventional exercise machines that work only one muscle group at a time, the special machines at Curves enable you to exercise *two* muscle groups at once. We call it the "double positive" workout. You're pushing with one muscle group and pulling with another. You work with greater intensity than normal, which helps keep your heart rate elevated. The Aerobic Recovery enables you to maintain your target heart rate while giving your muscles a rest. The end result is a lean, toned, strong, beautiful body. You get all of this in 30 minutes, three times a week. You'll just *look* like you spend all your time at the gym!

FUN: Walk into any Curves, and you will see relaxed, smiling, happy people working out at their own pace, listening to great music, and having a great time. It's a warm, supportive, no-stress atmosphere.

Although the Curves Workout is fast, you don't sacrifice safety. In fact, the Curves Workout is a very safe workout, primarily because you are pushing and pulling weight as opposed to lifting and lowering. The lowering of weight is called an "eccentric contraction" of the muscle. It's a much more difficult—and awkward—movement than lifting weight. It is responsible for 85 percent of all exercise injuries and is the cause of those sore muscles you feel after the standard "lift and lower" workout. Since you don't lower weight in the Curves Workout (you push and pull), you avoid the troublesome eccentric contraction. Another bonus: Most women do not feel any muscle soreness after a Curves Workout!

Another great feature of the Curves Workout is that you don't have to manage heavy weight stacks as you do at standard gyms. You can stop the exercise at any point and not get hurt by falling weights or an out-of-control machine. The Curves machines don't use weights; rather, they operate on hydraulic resistance—that is, when you push or pull the machine, you are actually moving fluid through a confined area. The faster you pull, the greater the resistance. You know how hard it is to run through water? The faster you try to run, the harder it gets. Even without using a weight stack, the Curves machines can give you a terrific workout. Similar to water exercise, hydraulic-resistance machines are very joint-friendly, but they are actually better than water exercise because on the machines, you can isolate individual muscle groups and create adequate resistance, which is difficult to do in water.

The Curves exercise machines enable you to work as hard as you want to work. They can accommodate the needs of newcomers but still challenge the needs of exercise pros.

The Curves Workout

The Curves circuit includes eight different machines arranged in a circle, or a circuit. You can join the circuit at any point (no waiting endless minutes for a vacant machine). There are Recovery Stations between each of the exercise machines. In the Curves Workout, you do as many repetitions as you can on each machine for 30 seconds. Then you move on to an Aerobic Recovery Station, where you give your muscles a rest while you maintain your target heart rate. You stay in the Recovery Station for 30 seconds and then go on to the next machine.

You begin with a three-minute warm-up period. You start on the circuit, but you work at a slower pace than you normally would as you warm up your muscles and get your heart rate up to target. (If you don't know what your target heart rate is, turn to pages 168–69.) After your warm-up, you work as hard as you can within your target heart rate. Check your heart rate every eight minutes during the workout. Go through the circuit three times, doing three repetitions of each exercise. For the last three minutes, slow down a bit to let your heart rate return to normal. After your cooldown, go over to the mat for three minutes of stretching.

The Curves Circuit

You can join the circuit at any point—the order of the exercises doesn't matter.

1 • **BICEPS/TRICEPS** • This machine works the biceps and the triceps.

   1. Sit firmly in the machine with your hands in a fist and your thumbs on top.

   2. Perform a full range of motion, but do not hit either the top or the bottom. Alternate, lifting one arm at a time. *Do not raise both arms at once. It can strain your back.*

RECOVERY STATION • 30 seconds

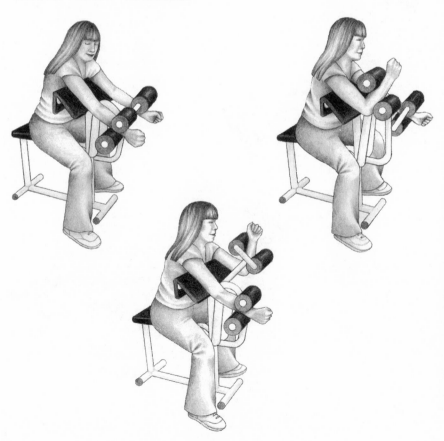

2 · LEG EXTENSION/LEG CURL · This machine works the quadriceps on the front of the thigh and the hamstrings on the back of the thigh.

1. Sit back on the machine and use the extra pad if necessary.
2. Place your ankles between the pads and extend your legs out almost straight, but do not hit.
3. Briskly bring your legs back until you almost touch the bottom of the machine.
4. Hold yourself in place with the handles.

RECOVERY STATION · 30 seconds

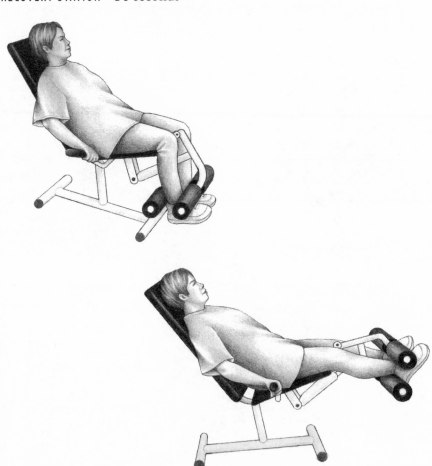

Exercises

3 • SHOULDER PRESS/LAT PULL • This machine works the trapezius, deltoids, and latissimus dorsi muscles.

1. Lean back, and grab the handles.
2. Start at shoulder height and lift until your arms are almost straight. Do not hit at either end. Move fast enough to create resistance, particularly in the pull-down motion.

RECOVERY STATION • 30 seconds

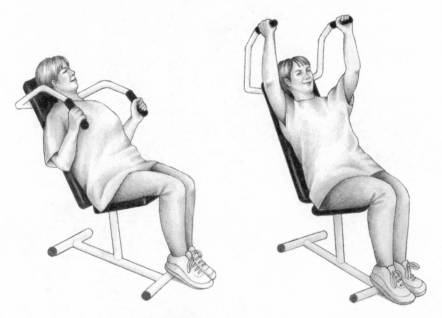

4 • HIP ABDUCTOR/ADDUCTOR • This machine works the hip adductor muscles of the inner thigh and the hip abductor muscles of the outer thigh.

Note: Enter and exit the machine from the center with the machine "legs" pulled apart. Do not enter from the side.

1. Sit back in the machine so that your back is supported, and brace yourself with the handles.
2. Place your legs in the pads and bring your legs together. Flex your toes toward the ceiling to prevent your knees from rotating. (Don't try to

conform to the bend of the leg bar. If your ankles are above the pad, it's okay.)

3. Extend your legs out as far and as comfortably as you can.

4. Bring your legs back to the center without their hitting each other.

RECOVERY STATION • 30 seconds

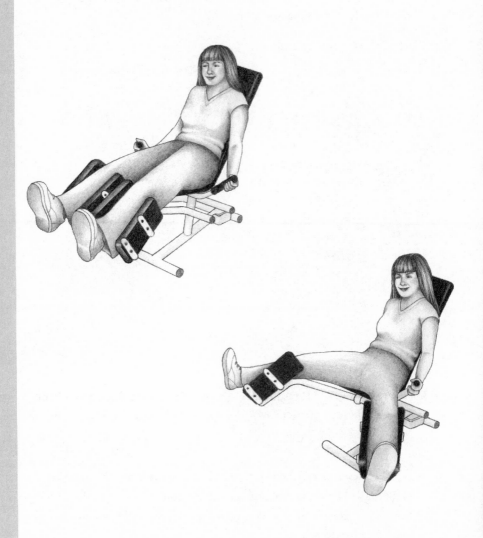

5 • **CHEST/BACK** • This machine works the pectoralis, rhomboid, and latissimus muscles.

1. Sit back in the machine and grab the handles at a point where they are midline of the muscles doing the work—about the height of your upper chest.
2. Push the handles forward, but do not lock your joints.
3. Bring the handles back to your starting position. Your body should stay firmly against the seat back. Lean back and work the chest and upper back muscles. This machine strengthens the muscles across the thoracic vertebrae (upper back).

RECOVERY STATION • 30 seconds

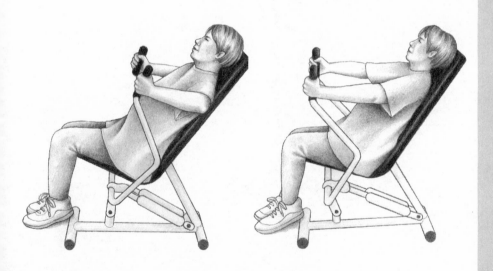

6 • **SQUAT** • This machine works the gluteus and quadriceps muscles.

Note: This machine requires extra caution. If you have back problems, begin with a small range of motion and by moving more slowly.

1. Stand straight on the edge of the platform and slowly lift the pads above your shoulders. Do not twist and bend to get into this machine. Step forward under the pads. Place your feet shoulder width apart and far enough forward so that your knees will not extend beyond your toes at the bottom of the movement.

2. As you squat, extend your buttocks backward while slightly arching your back.

3. Keep your eyes forward and come down until your thighs are parallel to the floor. Your knees should extend forward to your toes but not past them.

4. Go up quickly and come down slowly. Exhale as you come up.

RECOVERY STATION • 30 seconds

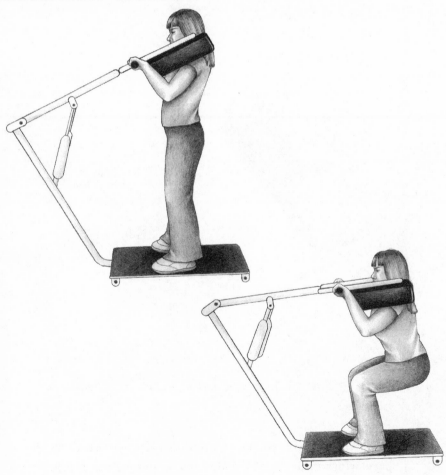

7 • **ABS/BACK** • This machine works the abdominals of the stomach and the spinae erector muscles of the lower back.

Note: If you have back problems, begin with a comfortable range of motion and take it slow.

1. Grab the handles with your arms straight.

2. Without moving your arms, curl forward, concentrating on the abdominal muscles doing the work. Exhale as you curl forward, but do not allow your head to go below your heart.

3. Curl back using your lower back muscles, and pull the bars backward until you are back against the seat. *Do not bend your arms.* This exercise works a very specific group of muscles with a very narrow range of motion.

RECOVERY STATION • 30 seconds

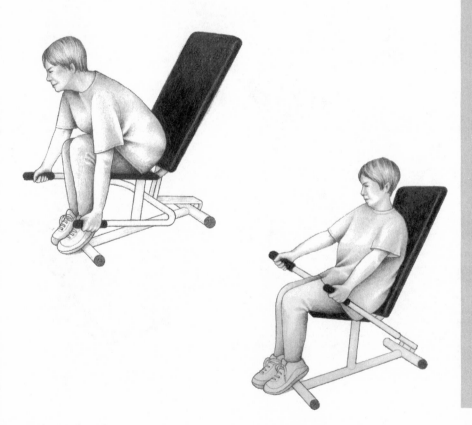

8 • LEG PRESS • This machine works the gluteus and quadriceps muscles.

1. Sit firmly in the machine. Place your feet at the top of the foot pad with your toes slightly over the top of the pad.
2. Push forward quickly until your legs are almost straight. Exhale as you push out.
3. Bring your feet back more slowly, as far as is comfortable. Let your knees go up rather than out to the side. Avoid moving rhythmically (to the music) or bouncing.

RECOVERY STATION • 30 seconds

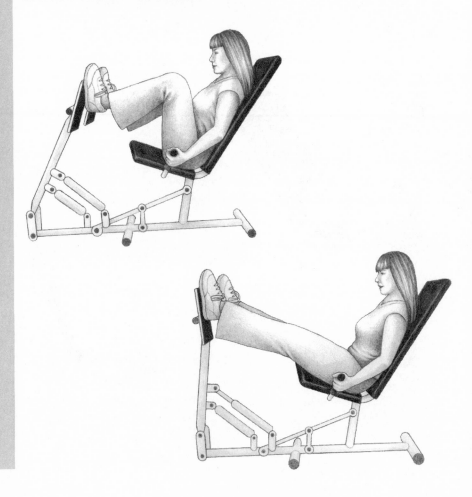

Gary's Tips for Newcomers:
How to Get the Most Out of Your Curves Workout

If you're just starting out at Curves, here are some things you should know that will help you maximize the benefit you are getting from your workout.

- **BE PATIENT** Don't try to work aggressively right away on every machine for the full 30 minutes. Start slowly and work your way up as you become stronger and more proficient on the machines.
- **BELIEVE IT** You need to believe that you can achieve the three components of the total workout—cardio and strength simultaneously, plus stretching, in just 30 minutes. If you don't believe it can be done, you won't take the time to learn the process or make the commitment to come in three times a week. Remember that there's a reason why 2 million women are Curves members and the number is growing exponentially each month.
- **STAY ON TARGET** Keep your heart in the target heart rate. Be sure to select the right target heart rate for you (check the chart on page 169). Don't fall below the target heart rate, because you won't get a good aerobic workout, but don't exceed it, because you'll wear yourself out too quickly. The reality is, as long as you're meeting enough resistance on the strength machines, and as long as your heart rate is elevated and sustained for 20 minutes, you're getting a cardio workout that's appropriate for your level. You don't have to kill yourself to get a great result.
- **LEARN THE RIGHT WAY TO LOWER YOUR HEART RATE** There are two ways to lower your heart rate while you are working out. One way is to simply move the machines more slowly, and that's what a lot of people do, but it's wrong. The problem is, you get your resistance from the speed of movement, so if you slow down too much, you're only moving at about 40 to 50 percent

of your true strength, which is not strength training. *Strength training requires that you move a resistance that is 60 to 80 percent of your maximum working ability.* You have to work your muscles harder than normal to make them stronger.

There's a better way to lower your target heart rate that doesn't jeopardize the effectiveness of your workout. You hesitate. When your heart rate is too high, when you move to the next machine, just sit there for five seconds and do nothing. Just wait. After the brief respite, you can once again move aggressively at the level at which you need to move to overload your muscles. You've just reduced the amount of work that you're doing by 16 percent—that's what five seconds out of the 30 seconds adds up to—and that will lower your heart rate very effectively. The good part is, your heart rate goes down without sacrificing strength training. Some of you may have to hesitate as much as 10 seconds before you begin to move aggressively, and that of course has reduced your work by one-third. Even that long a rest won't significantly alter your strength training. You're still moving six, seven, or eight repetitions of your exercise machine at a very heavy resistance so that you're still overloading the muscle. In contrast, if you did 12 repetitions at 40 percent of your maximum potential, you've done a good aerobic workout, but you're missing the strength training. Remember, strength training has probably been the missing link in your fitness program.

Gary's Tips for Curves Pros

- KEEP CHALLENGING YOURSELF As you become stronger, you need to work harder to maintain your muscle. Remember, if you don't work at 60 percent of your maximum ability, you will not get stronger, and you're not doing strength training, you are doing a purely aerobic workout. If you were doing eight to 10 repetitions on a given machine when you first started at Curves, you should now be up to 12 to 14 repetitions, and you should be working harder and harder. If the workout seems easy to you, it's because you're not exerting yourself enough. The machines are able to challenge anybody.

- **FINE-TUNE THE HESITATION METHOD** If you get on those machines and just blast, your heart rate will go up. If you need to lower your heart rate, but you don't want to lose the weight-training component of your workout, you will need to become very skilled at learning how and when to use the hesitation technique described earlier to bring your heart rate down.

- **THREE DAYS OF STRENGTH TRAINING IS ENOUGH** Many of our longtime members love to come to Curves and want to come every day. The problem is, when you strength train, you should take a day off between workouts to allow your muscles time to fully recover. There's a simple solution. Do your strength training Monday, Wednesday, and Friday, and do a purely aerobic workout on the other two days. You still go through the Curves circuit, but you work at half or less of your maximum ability. In other words, you take it easy on the machines, but you still keep your target heart rate elevated.

- **YOUR TARGET HEART RATE DOESN'T CHANGE** Many women mistakenly believe that they should keep increasing their target heart rate as they become more fit. This is wrong, and in fact, it can be dangerous. As you become more conditioned, you actually have to work *harder* to sustain your target heart rate. Your body has become accustomed to the extra workload and does not speed up as rapidly. Therefore, trying to exceed your target heart rate could put a strain on your heart.

TOTAL HEALTH SUPPLEMENTS FOR ENHANCING THE CURVES PROGRAM

When I travel around the country visiting Curves centers and talking to members, I am frequently asked the same two questions about nutritional supplements.

The first is, "If I eat a well-balanced diet, do I have to take supplements?" The second is, "If I take supplements, do I have to eat a well-balanced diet?"

The answer to both questions is "Yes!" I am a careful eater, but I also take a multivitamin with minerals and other important nutrients every day and recommend that you do too. In addition, I also take other supplements that can enhance health and prevent disease.

Many nutrition experts contend that supplements are useless and that everyone should get their vitamins and minerals from food. I think this is wishful thinking. I'm not suggesting that a pill can take the place of food. I'm a big proponent of good nutrition, and as you know, I believe that everyone should try to eat as healthy a diet as possible without making themselves crazy. The reality is, however, it's impossible to get all the nutrients you need from food alone. Fruits and vegetables are supposed to be a major source of vitamins and nutrients in our diet, but this is rarely the case. For one thing, few Americans eat enough of them (french fries don't count!). For another, modern farming practices have stripped the soil of the minerals that provide fruits, vegetables, and whole grains with important nutrients. Moreover, so-called "fresh" produce is rarely fresh. Typically, it is picked before it has been allowed to ripen, chilled to prevent spoilage, and then shipped thousands of miles away to neighborhood supermarkets, where it is then sprayed with a ripening agent. After all this abuse, it is sold to you. Produce that is picked prematurely does not contain as many vital nutrients as naturally ripened produce. Did you know that by the time a fresh orange finds its way to your home, it may contain virtually no vitamin C? This is assuming that you even eat oranges. How many times a day do you find yourself reaching for processed and convenience foods that are notoriously nutrient-deficient? How often do you eat dinner at a fast-food restaurant or skip lunch because you're pressed for time? Given our hectic schedules, we all do these things more often than we like to admit. The reality is, even if you are a very careful eater and are conscientious about eating healthy, fresh food, you will probably not be able to get enough nutrients from food alone.

Do not assume, however, that if you pop a vitamin pill daily you can forget about eating well. Even if fruits and vegetables are not as nutritious as they should be, they are still of great benefit. The fact is, food—especially fresh fruits and vegetables—contains hundreds of disease-fighting substances called phytochemicals (or phytonutrients). The handful of phytochemicals that have been scientifically studied have shown great promise for the prevention and treatment of chronic disease. And it's not just fruits and vegetables that are packed with important nutrients. Lean meat is a terrific source of protein and B vitamins, and it provides the best form of absorbable iron. Whole grains contain B vitamins and other important phytochemicals. No pill can duplicate the natural pharmacy found in whole foods. In summary, supplements are meant to work in tandem with food, not in place of it.

When you are on a weight-loss program, it is critical to maintain adequate nutrition *and* take your supplements. Subtle deficiencies in vitamins and minerals can contribute to food cravings, fatigue, mental confusion, and other problems that can undermine your weight-loss efforts. If you are tired all the time, you will not do your workouts. If you lack vitamins and minerals that help control blood sugar, you will be constantly hungry and tempted to cheat. If you catch a cold because you are not getting enough vitamins to keep your immune system strong, you will be less likely to exercise. Do you see how nutrient deficiency can sabotage your ability to lose fat and get fit?

How Much Is Enough?

Some people may be surprised to see that the Curves recommendations for the right doses of vitamins and minerals are higher than the Dietary Reference Intakes (DRIs) (formerly the RDAs) set by the National Academy of Sciences. For instance, the DRI for vitamin C is 60 milligrams for nonsmokers and 100 milligrams for smokers. At Curves, we recommend taking 1,000 milligrams of vitamin C daily. We're not alone in recommending higher doses than the DRI—in fact, most nutrition-oriented physicians agree with us. Why do we ignore the DRIs? Because they are hopelessly outdated.

There's a misconception among the public—and even among some members of the medical profession—about the purpose of the DRIs. The DRIs are not about maintaining optimal health, which is our goal, but about preventing specific deficiency diseases.

The DRIs are a revised version of the Recommended Dietary Allowances for vitamins and minerals, which were designed more than 50 years ago. The RDAs were the government's determination of the *bare minimum* amount of vitamins and minerals required to prevent a handful of diseases caused by gross nutrient deficiencies, such as scurvy (caused by a severe lack of vitamin C) and beriberi (caused by a severe deficiency in thiamine, a B vitamin). Although rare today in the Western world, these diseases are common in areas where there are frequent famines and food shortages. For example, during the 17th and 18th centuries, sailors confined to their ships for three to four months at a time without eating fresh fruits or vegetables frequently developed scurvy. An observant ship physician in the 18th century discovered that when sailors sucked on limes, they did not get scurvy, although he did not know why (that's why British sailors are nicknamed Limeys!). Today we know that just a tiny amount of vitamin C in your diet—10 milligrams daily—will eliminate the risk of scurvy. But just because you don't get scurvy doesn't mean that you are ingesting enough vitamin C to be healthy. In recent years, there has been a growing body of scientific evidence that shows that vitamins and minerals are not just needed to prevent rare deficiency diseases, but in fact they can help prevent and even reverse some of the more common diseases of the day, including heart disease, diabetes, cancer, cataracts, dementia, and birth defects. Notably, the doses of vitamins and minerals shown to have a beneficial effect are almost always higher than the DRIs.

- SAVE YOUR LIFE: A major population study found that people who consumed more than the DRI for vitamin C reduced their risk of dying prematurely by 60 percent.
- SAVE YOUR VISION: Women who took vitamin C supplements exceeding the RDIs were less likely to develop cataracts than those who did not.
- SAVE YOUR HEART: Men who consumed at least 300 milligrams of vitamin C daily had a 45 percent lower risk of heart disease than those who consumed less than 40 milligrams daily.
- SAVE FUTURE GENERATIONS: Test-tube studies show that it takes at least 200 milligrams of vitamin C to protect sperm from free-radical damage that could interfere with fertility and cause birth defects.

The dose recommendation for vitamin E is another example of how the DRI is outdated and outmoded. The DRI for vitamin E is 8 IU daily for women and 10 IU daily for men. Numerous studies—including several funded by the federal government—have demonstrated that vitamin E can enhance immune function, especially in older adults, and may protect against heart disease and Alzheimer's disease. In fact, in one study, high doses of vitamin E worked better than a commonly used prescription drug to slow the progress of Alzheimer's disease. Clearly, this vitamin has a protective effect on the brain and central nervous system. The problem is, it takes between 200 and 800 IU of vitamin E (depending on the problem) to achieve these beneficial effects. Given these new findings about vitamin E, it's inexplicable that the DRI is so low for this vital vitamin.

The argument that you can get enough vitamins from food alone doesn't hold water when it comes to vitamin E. In order to get at least 200 IU of vitamin E from food, you would need to eat more than 60 pounds of liver and 65 tablespoons of peanut oil daily. Isn't it easier to take a vitamin pill?

What's in a Good Multivitamin/Mineral Supplement?

The DRIs ignore the potential therapeutic effects of vitamins, minerals, and other nutrients, much the same way that most physicians ignore the importance of nutrition.

In contrast, the Curves recommendations are based on the latest studies on how to maximize the beneficial effects of individual nutrients. In fact, we even recommend taking some nutrients that are not even listed in the DRIs. The DRIs exclude whole categories of important nutrients that in recent years have been the subject of numerous research studies. For example, despite overwhelming scientific support demonstrating that a lack of essential fatty acids in the diet is responsible for a range of physical and psychological problems, there is no DRI for these nutrients. Nor is there a DRI for bioflavonoids, carotenoids, and other phytochemicals found in fruits and vegetables, which help maintain health and prevent disease.

There are key nutrients that everyone needs to maintain a strong, healthy body. You should make sure that your daily supplement regimen covers all the bases. Curves offers its own product line of high-quality supplements, including these nutrients, but I am providing you with the information you need to buy whatever product or combination of products is most convenient and economical for you.

Some of you with specific health concerns may need to take additional supplements. Please turn to Chapter 12, Special Health Concerns, for information on nutritional support for arthritis, adult-onset diabetes (type II diabetes), heart disease, pregnancy and postpartum recovery, premenstrual syndrome (PMS), osteoporosis, and menopausal symptoms.

Not all multivitamin and mineral supplements are equal. Many popular brands are based on the DRIs, and although they may contain a wide range of nutrients, they typically do not contain high enough doses to maximize health benefits. On pages 309–10, I provide you with a blueprint of what I feel should be in a good multivitamin, at the right doses. You can buy the Curves Complete Multivitamin and Mineral Formula at Curves, or you can purchase similar products at health-food stores, pharmacies, supermarkets, and discount drugstores. Read the labels. Some brands are not as complete as others. In many cases, you may need to buy more than one product to make sure that you are getting all the nutrients that you need in the right doses.

Before you purchase any supplements, I would like to tell you a bit about what's in a good multivitamin and why it's there.

Inside Your Multivitamin

Vitamins

Vitamins are organic substances that are essential for life and not produced by the body (except vitamin D), which means that you must get them from food and supplements. Vitamins include A, B-complex (B_1, thiamine; B_2, riboflavin; B_3, niacin; B_6, pyridoxine; and B_{12}, which contains cobalamin, biotin, and folic acid), C, D, E, and K. Vitamins A, D, E, and K are fat-soluble and are stored in fatty tissue. All vitamins are best absorbed with food, but it is particularly important to eat before taking fat-soluble vitamins. B-complex vitamins and vitamin C are water-soluble; what isn't used by your body is excreted in urine. It is best to divide up your dose of water-soluble vitamins and take them twice daily, in the morning and in the evening, for maximum absorption.

Water-soluble vitamins are measured in micrograms ($^1/_{1,000,000}$ of a gram), or a milligram ($^1/_{1,000}$ of a gram). Fat-soluble vitamins are measured in IUs (international units), with the exception of vitamin A, which is measured in REs, or retinol units. (RE and IU are interchangeable.)

Can you overdose on vitamins? Excessively high doses of some vitamins (well beyond what we recommend here) could, over time, cause problems. For example, vitamin B$_6$ in combination with folic acid can dramatically reduce your risk of developing heart disease. We recommend taking 40 milligrams of B$_6$ and 400 micrograms of folic acid. Yet extremely high doses of B$_6$—2 to 10 grams daily—can cause neurological problems. So even though we may recommend higher doses than the DRIs, it doesn't mean that the dose doesn't matter. Vitamins can be powerful medicines and should be treated with respect.

Minerals

Minerals (such as calcium, magnesium, and iron) are naturally occurring chemicals found throughout the body and must be constantly replenished through food and supplements. There are two kinds of minerals—*essential* minerals and *trace* minerals. Essential minerals must be consumed in greater quantity and are measured in milligrams or even grams. Trace minerals, which are required in minuscule amounts, are measured in micrograms and milligrams. You may be surprised to learn that even though only a tiny amount of trace minerals is needed by our bodies, they are of vital importance for our health. For example, chromium, a trace mineral, helps normalize blood sugar and insulin levels, which may help prevent insulin resistance and type II diabetes. Another trace mineral, selenium, may protect against many different forms of cancer and stroke. The more scientists study trace minerals, the more we realize how much the body needs them.

The Curves Complete Multivitamin and Mineral Formula contains more than 60 essential and trace minerals. I mention it here because I would like to clear up a point of confusion. Many people ask me why we include trace minerals such as lead and arsenic, which are reputed to be toxic. The answer is simple: We use only minerals from plant sources, not from heavy metals. In this form, these minerals are not toxic to the human body, and in fact are beneficial in that they help cleanse the body of toxic metals that we ingest from food and drugs. *A good multivitamin should contain an adequate amount of vitamins, essential minerals, and trace minerals.*

Antioxidants

Antioxidants are a family of hundreds of vitamins, minerals, and other nutrients that can be made by the body or found in food. Antioxidants are important because they protect our cells from damage inflicted by free radicals, unstable oxygen molecules that can damage healthy cells, which ultimately leads to heart disease, cancer, and premature aging. Although this explanation sounds very scientific, in reality we see the effect of free radicals in our everyday lives. For example, if you leave a cut-up apple in the open air, it will turn brown. Any cook worth her salt knows that if you sprinkle a few drops of lemon juice on the apple, it will stay fresh. Why? Lemon juice contains vitamin C, an important antioxidant. Our bodies are exposed to free radicals every day. In fact, you know those wrinkles and brown spots on your skin that drive you crazy? They are caused by ultraviolet light from the sun, which promotes the production of free radicals. Some of you may even be putting antioxidant creams on your face to slow down the aging process.

You may have heard of some of the better-known antioxidants, such as vitamins C and E, and the herb ginkgo biloba, which is well known as a brain booster. There are several other important antioxidants that are making headlines in scientific journals but that have not yet filtered down to the general public, including the following:

- COENZYME-Q10 (CO-Q10) may slow down the progression of neurological diseases and may prevent heart disease.
- ALPHA-LIPOIC ACID is a potent antioxidant that has been used in Europe for more than two decades to prevent and relieve complications associated with diabetes and may protect against brain aging.
- N-ACETYL CYSTEINE (NAC) can boost levels of glutathione, the body's primary antioxidant. Quercetin, found in onions and

garlic, helps maintain normal immune function and may
protect against cancer.

Eating an antioxidant-rich diet is important, but it is impossible to
get enough antioxidants from food alone. The better brands of high-
potency multivitamins include these and even other antioxidants. If
your multivitamin does not include Co-Q10, alpha-lipoic acid, and
NAC, at the very minimum, I recommend that you take an additional
antioxidant supplement. There are several good ones on the market
that also contain important phytonutrients, which are described below.

Phytochemicals (Phytonutrients)

Phytochemicals (also called phytonutrients) are chemicals that are found
in fruits and vegetables and that appear to have a protective effect
against many different diseases. Many are antioxidants. *A good multivitamin and mineral formula should contain key phytochemicals.* We include
several phytochemicals in our Curves Complete Multivitamin and Mineral Formula. For example, lutein, which is found in chopped spinach
and collard greens, is a member of the carotenoid family, a group of 500
different natural coloring agents that are found in plants. There is a high
concentration of lutein in the macula of the eye, and it's there for a reason. Recent studies show that lutein may help prevent macular degeneration, the leading cause of blindness among older women. We also
recommend taking lycopene, a carotenoid found in tomatoes and red
peppers, which may have a protective effect against breast, lung, and en-
dometrial cancers in women and prostate cancer in men.

Bioflavonoids are another important category of phytochemicals
that are ignored by the DRIs but are essential for health. Bioflavonoids
are found in citrus fruits, tea, berries, grapes, and pine bark. We include
mixed citrus bioflavonoids in our multivitamin, as do several other pre-
mium brands. Numerous studies have shown that bioflavonoids can
boost immune function, help prevent heart disease, and preserve mental function. They also enhance the effectiveness of vitamin C and
should be included in any supplement containing vitamin C.

Essential Fatty Acids

If you've been living on a low-calorie, low-fat diet, you are undoubtedly deficient in essential fatty acids. Essential fatty acids are called essential for a reason—they are needed everywhere in the body. The body uses two types of essential fatty acids: omega-6 and omega-3. Most people get enough omega-6 but are short in omega-3. Omega-3 fatty acids are converted into eicosapentenoic acid (EPA) and decosahexanoic acid (DHA). They are the major components of cell membranes, the protective covering around every cell, and are needed for the production of hormones. Recent studies show that essential fatty acids may help prevent many different forms of cancer, including breast cancer; help normalize bad blood lipids; and even relieve the aches and pains of arthritis. Many women find that essential fatty acids can reduce the discomfort of PMS. *If your multivitamin does not include essential fatty acids, you should take a fatty-acid supplement.*

Amino Acids

Amino acids are the building blocks of protein and of just about everything else in your body. Amino acids are essential for making muscle, but they are also needed for the health of your immune system, for the production of neurotransmitters in your brain that control your mood, and for repairing cells and tissues throughout your body. If you work out regularly, as you do on the Curves Weight-Loss and Fitness Program, your body may need additional amino acids to keep up with your increased activity. If you tire easily, take note: Amino-acid supplements may increase mental and physical stamina. Look for a multivitamin and mineral supplement that includes amino acids, or take a separate amino-acid supplement.

Tips on Taking Supplements

Multivitamins come in many forms, ranging from pills to capsules to liquid concentrates to powders. Use whichever products work best for you. High-potency multivitamin and mineral formulas are meant to be taken in two or more doses throughout the day for maximum absorption. To enhance absorption and avoid stomach upset, it's best to take your supplements with your meals unless told otherwise.

The FDA has label requirements for supplements, similar to the requirements for food labels. These new labels detail the quantity of the main supplement or supplements included in a product, in addition to a complete list of other ingredients.

Unless a label specifically says that you need to refrigerate a product, store your supplements in a cool, dry place, away from direct sunlight.

Women who are pregnant or who are breast-feeding should not take any supplements without first checking with their physicians. Your doctor will prescribe a special prenatal vitamin and mineral supplement designed for pregnancy. (In particular, pregnant women must not ingest more than 4,000 RE of vitamin A daily or they risk birth defects.)

Some supplements, notably vitamin E, essential fatty acids, and ginkgo biloba, are natural blood thinners. On the one hand, this is good because it helps prevent blood clots, which can cause a heart attack or stroke, but on the other hand, it can be problematic if you are undergoing surgery. If you are planning to have surgery, let your doctor know which supplements you are taking. You may have to discontinue taking some supplements a week or two before surgery.

Can you take supplements with prescription medication? In rare cases, a particular supplement may interact with a prescription medication. For instance, natural blood thinners (such as vitamin E, ginkgo biloba, and omega-3 fatty acids) may enhance the effect of prescription blood thinners. Some antioxidant supplements may negate the effect of chemotherapy drugs, which are designed to kill cells, not save them. If you are taking any prescription medication, check with your physician or pharmacist before taking a supplement to see if there could be an adverse interaction.

See pages 309–10 for a handy chart you can take with you to purchase your supplements.

Diet Pills: The Promise and the Hype

Some of you may have turned to this chapter thinking, *Great, here's where I find out about a magic pill that will melt the pounds away while I sleep!*

The fact is, you don't need diet pills to perform metabolic magic— that includes prescription and nonprescription. The Curves Weight-Loss and Fitness Program is the safest and most effective way to achieve your goals. Stick with the program, and the magic will happen.

Many of you have undoubtedly seen TV commercials for so-called natural diet pills that promise to burn off fat, or rev up your metabolism, or help you slim down overnight. There are two types of natural diet pills: metabolic stimulants and nonstimulants. Neither type of diet pill is a substitute for an effective diet and workout regimen. Metabolic stimulants, however, have proven health risks, and I believe they should be avoided. Nonstimulating supplements may be useful up to a point. Let me explain the difference between these two types of supplements.

As their name implies, metabolic stimulants contain stimulating chemicals such as caffeine and ephedra, a Chinese herb that contains amphetaminelike substances. These products do boost metabolism, but at a very steep price. They can cause a sharp increase in blood pressure, which can be quite dangerous for people with underlying heart conditions. There have been a few reported deaths from the use of metabolic stimulants. Even if they don't kill you, they can still make you jittery and promote insomnia. In addition, they may actually hamper your weight-loss efforts. Metabolic stimulants can trigger a rise in insulin levels, which will only aggravate carbohydrate cravings in carbohydrate-sensitive people. My advice: Don't use them. You don't need them.

Nonstimulating supplements may gently boost metabolism without the negative side effects. One herb often touted as a fat burner is hydroxy citric acid (HCA), synthesized from the rind of the garcina cambogia fruit, a pumpkin-shaped fruit popular in Asia. Some, but not all, studies have shown that HCA may slightly improve the results of a weight-loss diet. Minerals such as chromium and vanadium can help control blood sugar levels, which will help relieve food cravings in carbohydrate-addicted dieters. There are several combination weight-loss formulas on the market. If you choose to use a natural weight-loss supplement to support your efforts, please read the label carefully to make sure that it does not contain any stimulants. And don't be under the false impression that taking any pill is going to reduce the need to stick to your meal plan and do your workouts.

PART THREE

It's
About
Health

CHAPTER 12

SPECIAL HEALTH CONCERNS

The Curves Solutions for Arthritis, Diabetes, Heart Disease, Osteoporosis, Pregnancy, and Menopause

Curves is not just about looking great, it's about feeling your best and staying well. Regardless of your age, the Curves program can help you achieve optimal health so you can live a long, vital, and vigorous life.

Most chronic illness is not due to bad genes or bad luck: It's due to a careless lifestyle. If you eat poorly, don't get enough exercise, and are nutrient-depleted, your body will pay the price. In this chapter, I have written about different health challenges facing women, and I show how the basic principles of the Curves program can help a woman better manage a transition, such as pregnancy and menopause, or deal with a medical condition, such as heart disease or osteoporosis.

This information is not a substitute for good medical care, but it is certainly as important. It's also critical for you to get your annual physical examinations from your doctor, have regular mammograms after age 40, and call your doctor if you have a problem. It is equally important for you to take responsibility for your health and to adapt a proactive, healthy lifestyle.

Arthritis

As I write this section, *Time* magazine's cover story is, "The Coming Epidemic of Arthritis" (December 9, 2002). The word "epidemic" is not overstating the problem. There are currently 20 million people with osteoarthritis (the most common form), but by 2020 that number will double to 40 million as the baby-boom generation enters its 60s and 70s. In fact, 75 percent of all people over age 55 have some form of osteoarthritis, even if they don't feel any symptoms. I don't buy into the argument, however, that getting older automatically means that you have to become arthritic, and I don't think the fact that people are living longer is the sole reason we are seeing an increase in degenerative diseases in general and arthritis in particular. At the turn of the 20th century, serious forms of arthritis were rare in the United States, even among older people. Today, it is not uncommon for 40- and 50-year-olds to need knee surgery or even joint replacements. I believe that our modern lifestyle has played a role in exacerbating, if not creating, this epidemic. On the positive side, there is also compelling evidence that constructive changes in lifestyle can help spare your joints.

Arthritis is an umbrella term for more than 100 different diseases that involve inflammation of the joints. It can be mild—a minor ache or twinge now and then—or it can be so severe that you end up in a wheelchair. Arthritis can be caused by many unrelated factors, including autoimmune diseases such as lupus and rheumatoid arthritis, lyme disease, and even gout, a condition characterized by the deposit of uric acid crystals in the joints. The two most common forms of arthritis are osteoarthritis, caused by the degeneration of the joints due to wear and tear, and rheumatoid arthritis, which affects about 2.5 million Americans and strikes women three times more often than men.

Unlike osteoarthritis, rheumatoid arthritis is a systemic disease that in more severe cases can cause fatigue, fever, weight loss, and susceptibility to infection, and can even affect other organs within the body.

The major symptoms of rheumatoid arthritis include swelling, warmth, and redness in one or more joints, most often first striking the joints of the fingers and spreading to the wrists, knuckles, and knees.

Whatever the cause, arthritis can damage your joints—the spaces that connect bones. The end result of an arthritic condition is destruction of the articular cartilage, the unique substance that lines the joints, preventing bones from rubbing together. Articular cartilage is one of the wonders of nature. This thin, smooth but resilient lining of cartilage is what stands between you and pain. Articular cartilage allows the bones to move in a fluid fashion and protects the bones from excessive wear and force. As the cartilage wears down, the bones become more exposed, resulting in pain, stiffness, and swelling in the joints. As the joint space narrows and the destruction worsens, the joint lays down spurs of bone called osteophytes. Osteophytes are a mixed blessing. On one hand, they provide the joints with some stability by filling in the open spaces, but on the other, they can make joints feel stiff and creaky. Eventually, they can restrict movement and cause severe pain.

Although osteoarthritis can affect any joint, including those in the neck and spine, it is most likely to affect the weight-bearing joints of the lower limbs, notably the hip joints and knee joints. If your knee or hip feels stiff in the morning or stiffens up after sitting for a while, chances are you have a touch of arthritis.

For a disease that is nearly as common as the cold, we know very little about arthritis. We don't even know the precise cause. The conventional wisdom is that the longer you live, the more likely it is that your cartilage will wear out. But there are other factors at play. Genetics may play a role—for no apparent reason, some people are hit hard at an early age, while others can go well into their eighth and ninth decades with no problems. At any age, an injury that causes trauma to a joint can damage cartilage and cause arthritis. For example, runners and joggers who overtrain are prone to develop arthritis. If you jog or run, the forces exerted through your knees can be equivalent to more than 2,000 pounds of pressure. If you do this too vigorously or too often, your knees will give out. This is not to say that exercise is bad; in fact, being sedentary is a major risk factor for arthritis. You need strong muscles to support your joints, and if your muscles are weak, your joints will be forced to pick up the slack, and that can cause overuse injuries leading to arthritis. Free radicals, a culprit in virtually all chronic diseases, play a role in arthritis as well. Free radicals can attack the cells in cartilage, just like they attack cells all over the body, worsening joint inflammation and causing even more damage. That's why I want you to protect yourself by taking your antioxidant supplements!

Poor nutrition is another often-overlooked factor in arthritis. People who eat the standard sugar-laden, carbohydrate-rich diet are prone to have high levels of toxic chemicals called advanced glycation endproducts (AGEs) in their bodies. These chemicals promote free-radical production and inflammation. Subtle nutrient deficiencies can deplete the body of the resources it needs to keep free radicals in check, while at the same time hampering the body's ability to repair damaged cells and grow new cells.

There is no conventional cure for arthritis, and despite the best efforts of the pharmaceutical industry, no medication has been able to stimulate the growth of new cartilage. The standard approach is to reduce the pain, and the drugs of choice are nonsteroidal anti-inflammatory drugs (NSAIDs), either prescription or over-the-counter. Unfortunately, there are several side effects associated with the long-term use of NSAIDs, including gastrointestinal upset, which may lead to internal bleeding and even ulcers. NSAIDs may relieve symptoms, but they can also accelerate the destruction of cartilage.

There may not be a conventional cure for arthritis, but there are some highly effective natural therapies that not only relieve symptoms but may also stop and reverse arthritis.

The Curves Solution

LOSE EXCESS WEIGHT · Obesity is a major risk factor for arthritis for obvious reasons—the more weight your joints must support, the more likely they are to give out. Being overweight puts a tremendous strain on your hips, knees, and ankles. Studies have shown that even a relatively small reduction in weight can reduce your risk of developing osteoarthritis. Following the Curves Meal Plan will help you shed pounds safely and quickly.

EXERCISE · Here's what the Arthritis Foundation has to say about exercise: "Exercise reduces joint pain and stiffness, builds strong muscle around the joints, and increases flexibility and endurance." They recommend everything from walking to yoga to strength training to playing golf, as long as it gets you up and moving.

. . . BUT DO IT SAFELY · Those of you who can do a more intense workout should know that you shouldn't have to sacrifice your joints to be fit. You don't have to lift the heaviest weight at the gym or do hundreds of repetitions to maintain nicely toned muscles. A reasonably challenging regimen is all it takes to look and feel great. If you run or jog, don't do it every day. It will kill your knees. And don't spend the day on a step machine either, for the same reason. A recumbent stationary bicycle (in a reclining position) takes the stress off your knees and hips.

The best exercise regimen for your joints and your body is one that includes the three basic components I discuss in Chapter 9: stretching, resistance training, and aerobics. If you follow my suggested program, you will not be overworking any particular joint or muscle group. And please don't forget to stretch. Stretching helps maintain joint flexibility, which we lose with age. The loss of flexibility can seriously interfere with simple daily activities, such as trying to lift your arms over your head to put on a blouse or reaching for a dish in the cupboard. It can make you *feel* old before your time.

Do try Curves. The hydraulic-resistance equipment we use at Curves is very joint-friendly. It gives you a great workout without destroying your cartilage.

We'd love to see you at Curves, but if you have pain or are seriously arthritic, you may need to work first with a physical therapist or take a special exercise class for arthritic people. I urge you to embark on some form of regular physical activity. Water exercises are particularly soothing for people with aching joints, because water supports your body weight. Of course, talk to your doctor before starting a new exercise program. Even if you're in a wheelchair, you can do some moderate exercise that can help improve your range of motion and make you feel better.

NUTRITIONAL SUPPLEMENTS · Nutritional supplements provide the one bright light in the treatment of osteoarthritis. The combination of two supplements, glucosamine and chondroitin sulfate, works to relieve the pain and stiffness of arthritis while at the same time halting the production of enzymes that further destroy cartilage. In fact, the studies have been so convincing on glucosamine and chondroitin sulfate that many doctors are now telling their patients to try the combination. In some cases, this dynamic duo can also regenerate the growth of cartilage as long as the joint still has chondrocytes—cartilage-producing cells. Once the cells are destroyed, these supplements may still relieve pain, but they will not stimulate new cartilage growth. But there is no doubt that many people are feeling a lot better when taking these supplements. Unlike commercial painkillers that work immediately, it can take up to a month to feel relief with glucosamine and chondroitin sulfate. However, these supplements do not have nasty gastrointestinal side effects like commercial painkillers, and they appear to be safe even for long-term use. The usual dose is about 1,500 milligrams of glucosamine and 1,600 milligrams of chondroitin sulfate. You can divide your supplements into two to four doses and take them with your meals along with your multivitamin. Glucosamine and chondroitin sulfate are sold separately as well as in combination formulas. (We offer a combination formula at Curves.)

ESSENTIAL FATTY ACIDS · Good fats can reduce inflammation and relieve pain. If your multivitamin does not contain adequate essential fatty acids, do take a supplement.

Type II Diabetes

At the turn of the last century, diabetes was so rare that it ranked 100th in a list of diseases in the United States. Today, it is the sixth most common disease suffered by Americans and the seventh leading cause of death in the United States.

There are two types of diabetes, type I and type II. Type I diabetes is due to the inability of the pancreas to make enough insulin, the hormone that regulates blood-sugar levels. As discussed in Chapter 3, type II diabetes is not caused by too little insulin but rather by a loss of sensitivity to insulin, and it accounts for 90 percent of all cases of diabetes. Type II diabetics are insulin-resistant—that is, their pancreas is pumping out plenty of insulin, but their cells do not utilize it efficiently. Obesity is the major risk factor for developing type II diabetes and, along with diabetes, is an underlying cause of hyperinsulinemia, or too much insulin for too long.

By now you should know that a diet that is high in sugar-yielding carbohydrates—i.e., the standard American diet—is the primary reason why so many people are getting fat and becoming diabetic. Since 1900, our annual sugar consumption per person has gone from five pounds to 150 pounds. Our grains have been refined to the point that they are one step away from pure sugar. Important minerals that naturally helped maintain normal blood-sugar levels, such as chromium and magnesium, and fiber, which slows down the burning of carbohydrates, have been processed out of grains. What's left is an unhealthy, disease-promoting diet.

The first sign of type II diabetes is often elevated blood sugar, but that doesn't mean that diabetes is inevitable. Losing weight, reducing your sugar intake, increasing your intake of high-fiber foods, and starting an exercise program may keep diabetes at bay. In other words, you don't have to get this disease.

In a major study following the health and lifestyle of 84,941 female nurses from 1980 to 1996 (the famous Nurses' Study), researchers found a strong correlation between diabetes and a lack of exercise, a high intake of sugar and trans-fatty acids in the diet, and smoking. According to the study, "Overweight or obesity was the single most important predictor of diabetes." Interestingly, women who did not have an occasional alcoholic beverage (on average, half a drink per day) were also at an increased risk. (Even though alcohol is high in sugar, in limited quantities, it appears to offer significant health benefits.) By the way, even in the absence of obesity, a sedentary lifestyle greatly increased the risk of developing diabetes.

The standard prescribed diet for diabetics is the low-fat, high-carbohydrate diet that's also prescribed for heart patients. As noted earlier, many medical professionals are beginning to question the wisdom of giving people who already have elevated blood sugar more glucose-producing foods. We know that prediabetics do better by cutting down on simple carbohydrates and eating more lean protein, vegetables, and limited amounts of high-fiber whole grains and fruit that is low in sugar. It makes sense that diabetics should follow a similar diet. However, high-protein diets that allow unlimited protein can be dangerous for diabetics, who are prone to develop kidney problems. If you have diabetes, you must be under the care of a physician, preferably one who will not simply write out a prescription for a drug but also will help you incorporate a healing program of the right diet and exercise.

The real danger of diabetes is that it will lead to further problems down the road, such as heart disease, kidney disease, cataracts, nerve damage, and dementia. As discussed in the section on arthritis, chronically high levels of blood glucose can promote the formation of toxic AGEs, which in turn trigger inflammation and free radicals. If you have diabetes, you need to take care of yourself. Your lifestyle is what got you into this mess, and your lifestyle can help lift you out.

The Curves Solution

FOOD IS YOUR BEST MEDICINE • Cutting back on sugar-yielding carbohydrates will help restore insulin sensitivity. Fiber is your best friend! Try to eat about 30 grams of fiber daily. Slow-burning, high-fiber carbohydrates can help keep blood sugar under control. Ample amounts of protein (but not unlimited) and good fats are also important to keep your blood sugar normal. Find a smart, nutritionally oriented physician to help design the right diet for you.

EXERCISE • When it comes to metabolic disorders such as diabetes, exercise is a powerful tool for restoring normal insulin sensitivity. If you have above-normal blood-glucose levels, a regular exercise program can help restore normal blood-sugar levels. Exercise can also help improve blood circulation, which is often impaired in diabetics. Remember, obesity is the major risk factor for diabetes. If you need to lose weight, exercise is the only way to burn off the fat and keep it off.

EXERCISE SAFELY · If you've been diagnosed with diabetes, you should not embark on any exercise program unless you are under a doctor's supervision. If you are taking medication, you may need to take certain precautions before and during your workout. Be sure your doctor gives you specific information on how to exercise safely.

DON'T SMOKE · The combination of diabetes and smoking is deadly. Diabetics are prone to nerve damage, especially in their feet and legs, due to poor blood circulation. Your nerves are fed by small blood vessels. Since smoking further damages blood vessels, it can starve your nerves of vital nutrients, causing a condition called neuropathy. In severe cases, nerve damage can result in the amputation of a foot or limb. The bottom line: Don't smoke.

SUPPLEMENTS · If you have diabetes, you must check with your doctor before using any supplements. The following supplements have been found to be quite helpful for people with type II diabetes.

ANTIOXIDANTS: If you have high blood sugar, chances are your body is teeming with free radicals. Take a high-potency multivitamin/mineral supplement with the antioxidants I recommend in Chapter 11. One antioxidant in particular, alpha-lipoic acid, has been used safely in Europe for more than two decades to treat complications associated with diabetes, such as peripheral neuropathy. The usual dose is between 50 and 100 milligrams daily. If alpha-lipoic acid isn't in your multivitamin and if you are at risk of diabetes, consider taking it as a separate supplement.

CHROMIUM: Chromium, a trace mineral, enhances the activity of insulin in the body, thus reducing the amount of insulin required to control blood-sugar levels. According to the Human Research Nutrition Center at the U.S. Department of Agriculture, more than 50 percent of Americans are chromium-deficient. In one study, USDA researcher Richard Anderson, Ph.D., working with Chinese researchers at Beijing Hospital, tested the effect of chromium supplementation on patients diagnosed with type II diabetes. Within two months, patients given 100 micrograms of chromium twice daily showed significant improvement in blood-sugar levels. Be sure that your multivitamin/mineral supplement has chromium.

Heart Disease:
The Number-One Health Risk for Women

More than half a million women die annually from cardiovascular disease, diseases of the heart and blood vessels, such as heart attack and stroke. Cardiovascular disease is the number-one killer of both men and women in the Western world. Until midlife, men are at greater risk of having a cardiovascular disease than women, but once women reach menopause, they are equal partners in risk of falling prey to these diseases. In fact, women are nearly twice as likely to die from their first heart attack than men are. And don't assume that heart disease is just an *old* woman's problem. Twenty thousand women under age 65 die of heart attacks each year. I'm not telling you this to panic you—I'm telling you this because there's a great deal you can do to prevent this from happening to you.

Most heart attacks occur because the arteries delivering blood and oxygen to the heart become clogged with plaque—a thick, yellowish, waxy substance that consists of dead cells, cholesterol, and other debris. This condition is called atherosclerosis. Over time, the accumulation of plaque can narrow the arteries to the point that blood flow is seriously compromised, or a piece of plaque can lodge in the artery, which also blocks the flow of blood. If the heart does not get enough oxygen, heart cells begin to die. Sometimes women experience angina or chest pain, alerting them to this problem before they have a heart attack, but very often they don't.

If the carotid artery delivering blood to the brain becomes filled with plaque, it could cause a stroke, resulting in the death of brain cells. Some women have mini-strokes called "transient ischemic attacks" (TIAs) before they have a major stroke, but sometimes a stroke seems to come out of nowhere. Both conditions can be lethal if not caught in time and treated appropriately.

I have a particular interest in educating women about cardiovascular disease because I lost my mother to it. As I mentioned in Chapter 1, my mother died of a stroke at an early age, leaving behind five children. My mother suffered from high blood pressure, a risk factor for both heart disease and stroke. Although she was taking medication to lower her blood pressure, it did not cure her disease, and it barely controlled her symptoms. It simply masked them. I believe that when it comes to health, the best approach is one that gets to the root of the problem or, even better, prevents it from happening in the first place. I know that I can't rewrite my mother's history, but I can change the destiny of other women who may not be taking care of themselves as well as they should. The Curves Weight-Loss and Fitness Program can help prevent and reverse many of the risk factors leading up to cardiovascular disease. Every woman should know what these risk factors are and what she can do to prevent them.

Are You at Risk?

AGE · The older you are, the greater your risk of heart disease, simply because you are more likely to have one of the risk factors listed below.

FAMILY HISTORY · If your father had a heart attack before the age of 56, or your mother had one before the age of 60, you are at an increased risk of having one yourself. Please do not assume that this means that you will automatically develop heart disease. Genetics is just part of the story. If your parents smoked, were inactive, were overweight, or had other risk factors themselves, their heart problems might have nothing to do with you or your genes.

HAVE YOU GONE THROUGH MENOPAUSE? · As soon as a woman reaches menopause—even if it is surgically induced by a hysterectomy—her risk of heart disease increases with each passing year. Therefore, menopausal women need to be vigilant about maintaining their overall health and adopting a healthy lifestyle.

OBESITY · If you are 20 percent or more above your ideal weight, you are considered obese. Obesity increases the amount of work your heart has to do to pump blood throughout your body, therefore increasing your risk of having a heart attack or stroke.

HIGH LEVELS OF BLOOD LIPIDS · Do you have high cholesterol levels? Abnormally high levels of blood lipids are often a sign of atherosclerosis. At your annual physical, your doctor should check your cholesterol levels. Levels over 200 milligrams per deciliter may be considered too high, depending on other risk factors. Keep in mind that total cholesterol is not nearly as important as the kind of cholesterol you have. Good cholesterol, high-density lipoprotein (HDL), helps keep your arteries clear of plaque; therefore, high levels of HDL are good. You want to keep your HDL levels over 35. Bad cholesterol, low-density lipoprotein (LDL), can inflict significant damage on the arteries and promote the formation of plaque. You want to keep your LDL levels under 130.

The ratio of total cholesterol to HDL should not exceed six to one. Therefore, if your total cholesterol is 240, your HDL should be 40 or higher.

Your doctor should also measure your level of triglyceride, a type of fat that is found in the blood and can be measured by a simple blood test. Women who have triglycerides over 190 are at greater risk of heart disease.

Physicians often prescribe cholesterol-lowering drugs for high blood lipids. It's not my aim to come between you and your physician, but if you do decide to use drugs, I urge you to also combine dietary and lifestyle changes. You may find that making these changes reduces or even eliminates your need for drugs.

HIGH BLOOD PRESSURE · About 30 million women have high blood pressure—that is, blood pressure that is above the average 120/80. (Anywhere from 110/65 to 120/80 is considered normal. Blood pressure over 130/90 is often treated with medication to bring it down.) Although I favor natural remedies, if you are unwilling to control your high blood pressure through dietary changes, exercises, and supplements, then you should take medication. High blood pressure is often called the "silent killer" because very often women don't have any symptoms until they have a stroke or heart attack. Your family physician or your gynecologist should measure your blood pressure when you have your checkups. If you have high blood pressure, you must be monitored by your physician. *Do not let it go untreated.* Women with untreated high blood pressure run a greater risk of stroke, heart disease, atherosclerosis, aortic aneurysm (rupture of the aorta, the primary artery delivering blood to the heart), and kidney disease.

About 95 percent of all cases of high blood pressure are called essential or primary hypertension, and no one knows the cause. There is a strong link, however, between stress, anger, and hostility, and a tendency to develop high blood pressure. In my experience, many women with high blood pressure are often under undue stress or react badly to stress. Learning stress-management techniques and making exercise a regular part of your life can do wonders for these women.

DIABETES · Diabetic women are at double the risk of having a heart attack than nondiabetic women. Constant exposure to high levels of glucose and insulin can damage blood vessels. High insulin levels can also increase the risk of high blood pressure. Insulin causes the kidneys to maintain a higher sodium balance in the blood and, as a result, a higher blood volume. The higher the blood volume, the harder the heart has to work to pump it throughout the body. Many cases of type II diabetes can be prevented, if not controlled, by eating the kind of low-glucose-producing diet recommended in the Curves Meal Plan.

SEDENTARY LIFESTYLE · I have a vested interest in getting you to exercise, so don't take my word for it—listen to the American Heart Association. They list physical inactivity as a serious risk factor for heart disease, right up there with high cholesterol!

SMOKING · Smoking does particularly nasty things to a woman's cardiovascular system. With every puff of smoke, you are inhaling hundreds of toxic free radicals that go on a search-and-destroy mission in your body, often targeting healthy cells. In addition, smoking makes a woman's blood more likely to develop blood clots, which become lodged in an artery, blocking the flow of blood. And while I'm on the subject, lung cancer, not breast cancer, is the number-one cancer killer of women. And what is the chief cause of lung cancer? Smoking.

THE LETHAL COMBO: BIRTH CONTROL PILLS AND SMOKING · Estrogen increases the level of fibrinogen, a substance in the blood that promotes clotting. By itself, it's a small risk, but when combined with cigarettes, which do the same thing, it can be lethal. In fact, women who smoke and take the pill have up to a 40 percent increase in their risk of developing cardiovascular disease.

STRESS · Though not a proven risk factor, many scientists hypothesize that stress could be a hidden risk factor for heart disease. When people are under constant stress, they produce hormones that raise their heart rate and their blood pressure, forcing their hearts to work harder. To compound the problem, stress hormones also send blood insulin levels soaring, which in itself can damage arteries.

Only the first three risk factors on this list, your age, your family history, and whether or not you have gone through menopause, are beyond your control. There is an overwhelming amount of evidence showing that simple changes in diet, exercise, stress reduction, and even taking nutritional supplements can tip the odds in your favor.

The Curves Solution

CLEAN UP YOUR DIET · If you follow my dietary recommendations in Chapter 7, Nutrition for a Great Body, you will be eating a heart-healthy diet. Here are some of the main points.

- Keep your fat intake to 30 percent or less of your daily calories, and stick to healthy fats. Cut out the trans-fatty acids—that means don't eat margarine, and avoid processed baked goods and foods that contain trans-fats.
- Watch your intake of saturated fat—eat low-fat or no-fat dairy products and lean cuts of meat. Use butter sparingly, but it's better than margarine.
- Olive oil is best for cooking. Do as the Italians do. Dip your bread in olive oil instead of using butter or margarine.
- Eat fish—omega-3 fatty acids are good for your heart.
- Fill your plate with fruits and vegetables. These foods contain flavonoids and other phytochemicals that are great for your heart.
- Reduce your intake of glucose-producing foods that bathe your body in high levels of insulin. Avoid bleached, processed flour. Stick to whole grains in moderate amounts.
- If you are salt-sensitive, don't add it to your food. It could raise your blood pressure.
- More than one glass of alcohol daily may increase a woman's risk of heart disease.

Tap the Power of Antioxidants

Your high-potency multivitamin and mineral supplement should contain adequate antioxidants to protect the cells in your arteries from free-radical damage. Here are some of the ways that antioxidants help to keep your cardiovascular system strong.

CO-Q10 More than 50 studies confirm that Co-Q10 is good for your heart. It's been used in Europe for decades to treat heart failure, and knowledgeable physicians are beginning to recommend it to their patients in the United States. Co-Q10 performs two important jobs in the body. First, it's a powerful antioxidant. Second, it helps cells make energy, the fuel that runs the body. Energy is created in our cells by microscopic structures called mitochondria. Co-Q10 is essential for energy production. Rich in mitochondria, the heart is one of the most energy-dependent organs in the body. Without proper energy, the heart cannot pump efficiently, which could lead to heart failure.

VITAMIN C A major study of 12,000 men showed that those with the highest intake of vitamin C lived longer and had a significantly lower risk of heart disease. (Sorry, they did not include women in the test!) Vitamin C works with vitamin E in the body to prevent the oxidation (free-radical attack) of healthy cells.

VITAMIN E The amount of research showing that vitamin E can help reduce the risk of heart disease is overwhelming. Numerous studies confirm that it protects LDL cholesterol from oxidation, or free-radical attack, the primary cause of atherosclerosis. In a study of nearly 85,000 nurses, those who took vitamin E supplements for more than two years had a 41 percent lower risk of developing major heart disease than those who did not. Vitamin E may be of even greater benefit to people with existing heart disease. Consider the results of the Cambridge Heart Antioxidant Study, involving 2,002 patients with diagnosed heart disease, more than a third of whom had serious heart disease. Half the patients were given either 400 IU or 800 IU of vitamin E daily; the rest were given a placebo. In less than a year and a half, the researchers found that the group that took vitamin E had 77 percent fewer heart attacks than those who didn't. The results were so good that the researchers discontinued the study and gave everyone vitamin E.

Why wait until you have heart disease? Get the benefits of vitamin E now.

B VITAMINS LOWER HOMOCYSTEINE · Homocysteine is a protein produced by the body. In excess, it can increase the risk of heart disease, cancer, and Alzheimer's disease. How do you keep homocysteine in check? Make sure your multivitamin includes the B-complex vitamins.

EXERCISE YOUR HEART · Exercise is a powerful tool for preventing and reversing heart disease. It is also an underutilized tool. Half of all women lead sedentary lives, which, as noted earlier, increases the risk of developing heart disease as much as high cholesterol does. In fact, exercise can help normalize high cholesterol and boost levels of HDL (good cholesterol). If doctors handed out as many prescriptions for exercise as they do for drugs, I am confident we could eliminate most cases of heart disease!

It doesn't take much exercise for a woman to reduce her risk of having a heart attack. Just a half-hour a day of walking briskly for five days a week can cut a woman's risk of heart disease and stroke by 50 percent!

Exercise is a great stress reliever. It helps turn off stress hormones, but at the same time it conditions your heart to cope with stress in a more constructive way. Your body responds to the physical stress of exercise by constricting your blood vessels and increasing your heart rate, which is precisely what it does when it's under emotional stress. The difference is, when you exercise, you can control the situation. If you are vigilant about keeping your heart rate within your target zone, you can teach your body the right way to deal with stress without overreacting and overtaxing your heart. After you have been exercising for a while, you will find that you do not react as strongly when you are confronted with daily stressors, and the minor annoyances that once set off your stress hormones now don't seem to get to you.

Following the Curves Weight-Loss and Fitness Program will significantly reduce your risk of heart disease while at the same time trimming and toning your body. Remember, your heart is also a muscle, and any program that builds muscle will also benefit your heart.

Exercise can be of great benefit to women who already have heart disease and high blood pressure, as long as it is done correctly and under a doctor's supervision. If you have a heart condition or high blood pressure, talk to your doctor before starting an exercise regimen.

If you have high blood pressure, please start out slowly. Initially, keep your target heart rate at 50 percent of your maximum heart rate. Gradually increase your pace, and don't be in a hurry. As I noted earlier, small steps will still get you where you want to go. Take time out to enjoy the journey along the way.

Menopause: Natural Solutions

Before I tell you what menopause is, let me tell you what it isn't. Menopause is not a disease, it's not an ailment, and it's not the beginning of a downward spiral to old age and infirmity. If you don't believe me, go to your local Curves and check out the women in their fifties, sixties, and many even older, who are zipping through the workout with as much zest and endurance as their younger counterparts.

The official definition of menopause is the last menstrual period, but in fact, the hormonal changes leading up to menopause (known as perimenopause) may begin a full decade before menopause. The end of menstruation is due to the decreased production of sex hormones by the ovaries. As the body undergoes this transition—and sometimes for years after—women may experience symptoms such as hot flashes, night sweats, insomnia, depression, irritability, palpitations, vaginal dryness, anxiety, poor memory, and difficulty concentrating. After menopause, the adrenal glands should take over the production of sex hormones, at least enough to restore balance to the body, but that doesn't always happen as quickly or effectively as it should. If women are under a great deal of stress or are poorly nourished, their adrenal glands may not have enough reserve to assume this important task.

Postmenopausal women may develop specific health problems that need to be addressed. Osteoporosis is one of them, and I urge you to read the section on osteoporosis on pages 239–43. After menopause, women are also at much greater risk of heart disease, and all women should read the section on heart health on pages 226–34.

For the past 30 years, doctors have prescribed synthetic hormones— hormone-replacement therapy—for millions of menopausal women. By boosting levels of estrogen back to more youthful levels, HRT can help relieve menopausal symptoms. Short-term studies also suggested that there were widespread health benefits of taking hormones—notably, supplemental estrogen could stop the loss of bone that leads to osteoporosis, reduce the incidence of heart disease, and improve mood and memory in menopausal women. Although originally prescribed to relieve short-term menopausal symptoms, some women felt so good on HRT that they wanted to stay on it for their entire lives.

As I am writing this book, there is widespread fear and confusion in the United States about the use of hormone-replacement therapy for menopausal women. The Woman's Health Initiative, a major long-term study involving 16,000 women on HRT, recently reported that women who took a combination synthetic estrogen and progestin pill for more than five years were at a 29 percent greater risk of having a heart attack than women taking a placebo and at a 40 percent greater risk for stroke. Moreover, women taking HRT for more than five years were at a 26 percent increased risk of developing breast cancer. In fact, the researchers were so alarmed at these findings that they abruptly discontinued the study.

That left the 8 million postmenopausal women in the United States already taking synthetic hormones in a real quandary: Should they discontinue taking HRT and risk the return of unpleasant menopausal symptoms, or should they stay on HRT, even though it could increase their risk of getting sick?

I'm here to offer a third and better alternative: The Curves Solution. We don't feel that women should have to make a choice between feeling good and having good health. There are safer, natural remedies that can ease a woman's transition through menopause and at the same time help her strengthen her body and prevent disease. It's possible for menopausal women to have it all without risking their lives.

The Curves Solution

REVITALIZE YOUR ADRENAL GLANDS · If your body is not adjusting to menopause, it could be a sign of weakened adrenal glands due to excess stress. I know that modern life today can be tough, especially for women torn between jobs and kids or other family responsibilities. And I understand that you can't get rid of the stressors in your life, but you can try to fortify yourself so that they are not as damaging.

Exercise is a great stress reliever and mood elevator. When you are under stress, your adrenal glands are pumping out high levels of stress hormones, also known as "fight or flight" hormones. These hormones were designed to help our prehistoric ancestors flee from wild animals or hostile invaders. Today, they just accumulate in our bodies, making us feel edgy and even depressed. The best way to get rid of stress hormones is to burn them off with vigorous exercise, as nature intended you to do. Regular exercise not only controls stress hormones but also replaces them with mood-elevating hormones called "endorphins." Numerous studies have documented that people who suffer from anxiety and depression nearly always improve when they exercise regularly.

Don't forget to feed your adrenal glands the right food—high-quality protein and high-fiber carbohydrates. The wrong diet can be very taxing on your adrenal glands. In Chapter 2, I described how bombarding your body with glucose-producing carbohydrates causes a sudden drop in blood-sugar levels, which could trigger the release of stress hormones. If you are constantly on sugar overload, your adrenal glands will pay the price—and ultimately so will you, when you reach menopause.

Be sure to take a multivitamin containing B vitamins, which are natural stress relievers, including vitamins B_6, B_{12}, and pantothenic acid.

PHYTOESTROGENS · Some foods contain naturally estrogenic compounds that can help relieve menopausal symptoms such as hot flashes and night sweats. Phytoestrogens bind to estrogen-receptor sites on cells, thereby reducing the body's need for real estrogen. In particular, nuts and flaxseeds contain high amounts of phytoestrogens. You can purchase flaxseeds at most health-food stores and sprinkle a tablespoon or two in yogurt, salad, or even on cereal.

Soy foods are particularly rich in isoflavones, natural estrogenlike chemicals that appear to mimic the role of estrogen in the body. Tofu and soy protein are good sources of isoflavones. You can also take isoflavones in supplement form, and isoflavones are often included in special supplement formulas designed to relieve menopausal symptoms.

PROTECT YOUR BONES • Once a woman reaches menopause, she should take 1,500 milligrams of calcium daily in the form of calcium citrate and calcium malate, along with the right minerals to enhance bone formation and 400 IU of vitamin D. For more information about osteoporosis, see pages 239–43.

STAY FLEXIBLE • Postmenopausal women frequently complain of stiff, aching joints. You can relieve your symptoms and maintain your flexibility by doing the stretching exercises recommended in Chapter 9. Remember, the more sedentary you become, the more you will hurt.

TARGETED SUPPLEMENTS • There are several nutritional supplements that may help reduce menopausal symptoms and improve your physical and mental well-being. They can be purchased separately or found in a combination formula designed specially for menopausal women.

BLACK COHOSH • Black cohosh is an herb that is a time-honored remedy for women's ailments, including menstrual problems and menopausal symptoms. Your great-great-grandmother may have taken it in a popular herbal elixir for "women's complaints." Recently, the American College of Obstetricians and Gynecologists finally conceded what women have known for more than a century: Black cohosh can help relieve hot flashes. There have been several short-term studies on the use of black cohosh for menopause, and most have yielded positive results. In fact, the federally funded National Center for Complementary and Alternative Medicine at the National Institutes of Health is now funding a rigorous 12-month scientific study of black cohosh to determine its effect on hot flashes and other symptoms of menopause, and they report that the preliminary results are "encouraging." No one knows exactly how black cohosh works, but scientists recently discovered that it contains estrogenic compounds. It appears to have phytoestrogenic properties, but it may also work in other ways that have yet to be discovered. Black cohosh has been approved by the German Commission E, the scientific body that evaluates herbal therapies (like our FDA), as a treatment for menopause, PMS, and painful menstruation. The German Commission E is highly respected by the medical establishment, which makes this endorsement all the more powerful.

DONG QUAI · For centuries, Chinese herbalists have prescribed dong quai along with other herbs to treat the symptoms of menopause and bad menstrual cramps. A study conducted by Kaiser Permanente showed that taking 4.5 grams of dong quai daily over a six-month period did not relieve hot flashes any better than a placebo. Those of us who know something about herbal medicine were not surprised. Although dong quai has estrogenlike compounds, it has never been used by itself to treat menopausal symptoms. We have to assume that herbalists knew what they were doing when they combined it with other herbs. This herb works best when it is part of a combination herbal formula for menopause symptoms, not as a stand-alone herb. Dong quai also contains antispasmodic compounds that can help relieve menstrual cramps.

LICORICE · The same herb that we use in the west to flavor candy is highly esteemed in China for its medicinal properties. Why do I recommend this herb for menopause? Licorice can revitalize sluggish adrenal glands, coaxing the adrenals to do their part to make up for the missing estrogen. Moreover, licorice contains estrogenlike compounds that may also help relieve menopausal symptoms. In addition, licorice contains anti-inflammatory compounds that can relieve arthritis symptoms and ulcers. The one downside: Licorice can raise blood pressure, so if you have high blood pressure or a kidney condition, you should not use this herb unless you are under the supervision of a medical professional or knowledgeable healer.

RED RASPBERRY · Since ancient times, the leaves of the red raspberry plant have been brewed into a tea to help prepare the uterus for delivery. Although we don't know the precise mechanism, raspberry contains compounds that relax the smooth muscles of the uterus.

Osteoporosis: Standing Straight and Strong

About half of all women over age 65 have osteoporosis, the thinning and wearing away of bone, which in turn increases the risk of bone fractures or breaks. The problem begins much earlier in life, so don't assume that if you're in your 20s or 30s you don't need to know about this. The earlier you begin taking steps to prevent this problem, the better your chance of avoiding it.

The gradual loss of bone is a normal part of the aging process and happens to both men and women. Osteoporosis, however, is caused by the accelerated loss of bone. Women are four times more likely than men to get osteoporosis, for two reasons: First, since women are smaller, they have less bone mass to begin with, so they feel the loss of bone more acutely. Second, the loss of estrogen after menopause accelerates bone loss in women.

Your genes and personal habits may be working against you. Slender, small-boned Asian and Caucasian women are at the greatest risk of developing osteoporosis. Women who smoke or who drink more than two glasses of alcohol daily are also at a heightened risk. Osteoporosis is responsible for about 1.5 million fractures each year, mostly in the hip, spine, and wrist. About 40 percent of all postmenopausal women will develop vertebral fractures that result in the rounded back or dowager's hump. Osteoporosis is not just a cosmetic problem—it can be deadly. Out of the 300,000 women each year who get hip fractures, 20 percent die from complications such as pneumonia or blood clots within six months of their injury. In severe cases, women with osteoporosis are so frail that everyday activities such as stooping down to hug your grandchild or picking up a grocery bag can cause bones to break. Osteoporosis can shorten your life and ruin your lifestyle.

The good news is, osteoporosis can be prevented, and even if you have been diagnosed with it, its progression can be slowed down with the right treatment.

In order to understand how to prevent and treat osteoporosis, you need to know how bone is made in your body. Bone consists of several minerals, including a high amount of calcium and phosphorus salts, and small amounts of trace minerals such as zinc, magnesium, iodide, and fluoride. (Now can you see why trace minerals are so important?) Throughout our lives, our bones undergo a continuous process called "remodeling," in which old bone is broken down and new bone is created in its place. Osteoblasts are cells that make new bone. Osteoclasts are cells that break down old bone. When we are young, the bone-making cells outpace the bone-breaking cells. After age 35, men and women begin to lose about 1 percent of their bone mass each year, but after menopause, women lose between 2 and 4 percent of their bone mass over the course of the next decade.

The high rate of osteoporosis among postmenopausal women is due to the diminished production of estrogen by the ovaries. Estrogen is essential for the absorption of calcium by the bones and is needed for bone growth. In fact, the one proven benefit of estrogen-replacement therapy is that it can halt the loss of bone after menopause. It doesn't, however, stimulate the growth of new bone. And many women are reluctant to take estrogen because it increases the risk of breast cancer and heart disease.

So what's a woman to do? Fortunately, there are safe and natural strategies to prevent and treat osteoporosis, and every woman needs to know about them.

The Curves Solution

GET A BONE-DENSITY TEST · By age 40, all women should have a baseline bone-density test. Ask your family physician or gynecologist about it. In some cases, it can be done right in your doctor's office. If your bone density is less than 85 percent of what it should be at your age, your doctor may recommend medication to stem further loss. There are several new drugs on the market—they all have some unpleasant side effects, but some women may have to take them. You can also try to incorporate some of the natural therapies listed below to help reverse bone loss.

FEED YOUR BONES · Your bone-making cells need the right raw materials so they can make new bone. In particular, they need enough calcium and other minerals on hand to do their job. All women should take a supplement of 1,000 to 1,500 grams of calcium daily, as well as 400 IU of vitamin D, which is needed to absorb calcium and other minerals. It's critical for teenage girls and women in their 20s to consume adequate calcium so they can create a strong, dense bone mass during their peak bone-making years. Likewise, it is essential for postmenopausal women to consume enough calcium to counteract the loss of estrogen. Good food sources of calcium include dairy products, broccoli, kale, and canned salmon with bones (don't get boneless—the calcium's in the bones!).

Unfortunately, according to the FDA, most women get only half the calcium they need daily from food, if that much. What happens if you don't have enough calcium? Most of the calcium in your body ends up in your teeth and bones, but calcium plays a critical role in a number of vital body functions, such as muscle contraction (including the beating of your heart), blood clotting, and nerve transmission. If you don't maintain an adequate calcium supply, your body will sap calcium from your bones to use for other tasks. This doesn't leave your bone cells with enough material to make new bone.

Can taking calcium supplements really make a difference? Let me tell you about a double-blind, placebo-controlled study conducted at the University of California involving 59 postmenopausal women. The women were divided up into four different treatment groups. One group was given a 1,000-milligram calcium supplement daily. The second group was given a mineral formula containing 25 milligrams of zinc, 5 milligrams of manganese, 2.5 milligrams of copper, and no calcium. The third group was given a combination formula containing 1,000 milligrams of calcium citrate and calcium malate, plus the mineral formula with zinc, manganese, and copper. The fourth group was given a placebo (or sugar pill). Women who took the placebo experienced a 3.25 percent loss of bone mass over a two-year period, which demonstrates what happens when you don't take anything. Those taking the minerals alone showed 1.89 percent bone loss, which is better than doing nothing, but not much better. Those taking calcium alone had a 1.25 percent loss of bone mass, which still put them in the minus column. Amazingly, the women who took the calcium-mineral combination had a *1.48 percent increase* in bone mass—that's right, I said *increase*. Clearly, taking the right combination of calcium and minerals can make a big difference in whether you lose or gain bone mass and, ultimately, whether you get osteoporosis. Not all forms of calcium are well absorbed by the body. Calcium citrate and malate are more expensive than calcium carbonate, but they are better absorbed.

CONSIDER TAKING IPRIFLAVONE · Ipriflavone is a synthetic version of a phytochemical found in soybeans. Similar to estrogen, it appears to halt the loss of bone after menopause. It should be taken with calcium to get maximum benefit. In a study conducted in Italy, women who took 200 milligrams of ipriflavone three times daily, along with 1,000 milligrams of calcium, did not have any bone loss in their spine, whereas women who took only calcium had 4.9 percent loss after two years. (They were not taking minerals with their calcium!) Ipriflavone is sold separately and is included in combination formulas designed for bone health and/or menopause.

EXERCISE · Here's yet another reason to begin taking exercise seriously. The right exercise is not only good for your muscles, but it can also help save your bones. The combination of weight-bearing exercises (walking, running, and jogging) and resistance training can help strengthen existing bone and stimulate the formation of new bone. In addition, exercise can help maintain stability and balance, which makes it less likely that you will fall and break a bone.

CAUTION · If you are frail or prone to fractures, or if you have been diagnosed with osteoporosis, talk to your physician before embarking on an exercise regimen. Although the right exercise can be extremely helpful, the wrong exercise (high-impact aerobics or movements like twisting from your spine) may aggravate your condition.

PLANT ESTROGENS (PHYTOESTROGENS) · Phytoestrogens, particularly those found in soy foods, may help improve calcium absorption in the body. Several studies have shown that the mildly estrogenlike compounds in soy products can help reduce bone loss and improve calcium retention.

CURVES TIP • The Curves soy protein shake that many of our members drink daily is a great way to get beneficial phytoestrogens. If you mix it with eight ounces of skim or low-fat milk, you can add up to 300 milligrams of calcium to your daily intake.

Pregnancy: Staying Fit

Pregnancy is a critical time in a woman's life, when she needs to focus on her health for two important reasons: her baby and herself. First, healthy moms are more likely to give birth to healthy babies. Second, a woman who ignores her own needs during pregnancy can be setting herself up for a lifetime of chronic illness.

It's particularly important to pay attention to the amount of weight you gain during pregnancy. All women will need to put on some extra pounds to nourish the growing baby. The mother must not only provide for the increased demands that pregnancy places on her body, but she must also make sure that her baby is getting enough nutrients to develop normally. *Pregnancy is not the time to go on a weight-loss diet. It is the time to eat a diet that's as healthy and nutrient-rich as possible.*

Your doctor will help you determine how much weight you should gain during pregnancy, but there are some standard guidelines.

- Normal-weight women should gain between 25 and 35 pounds.
- Underweight women should gain between 28 and 40 pounds.
- Overweight women should gain between 15 and 25 pounds.

Gaining too little weight can increase the risk of premature birth. Gaining too much weight can increase the risk of gestational diabetes, which is dangerous for both mothers and babies.

There's yet another reason to be concerned about exceeding the weight guidelines during pregnancy—the more you gain, the harder it will be to take it off after delivery. In fact, a recent NIH study found that excessive weight gain during pregnancy is now a major contributor to the obesity epidemic in the United States. Researchers monitored 577 pregnant women from early pregnancy through the first year after they gave birth. Out of this group, 40 percent of them gained more than the recommended weight during pregnancy, and 25 percent were at least 10 pounds heavier a year after giving birth. The study concluded that women who gained too much weight during pregnancy were *four times more likely to be obese* one year after giving birth than mothers who stayed within the recommended weight gain.

In another study on pregnancy and weight gain, researchers found that women who gain more than the recommended weight during pregnancy—and fail to take it off in a timely fashion—are at a much higher risk of being obese nearly a decade later.

Pregnancy should not condemn you to a lifetime of obesity. There are simple things that you can do to stay fit and trim, and still provide your baby with the nutrition he or she needs to grow healthfully and normally.

The Curves Solution

EAT WELL · Good nutrition is the cornerstone of a good pregnancy and a great postpartum recovery. Pregnant women need to eat on average an additional 300 calories daily. Make every calorie count, particularly in the first trimester. Many women gain weight rapidly in the beginning by loading up on fattening, low-nutrient junk food, which can cause unnecessary weight gain. A better approach is to pace yourself so you gain slowly and steadily over the entire nine months. If you gain the right amount of weight during pregnancy, chances are you will lose it after delivery and be back to your normal size within six to nine months postpartum.

Ideally, you want to gain two to five pounds the first trimester, and a pound a week, or three to four pounds a month thereafter, until delivery.

Your doctor will prescribe a prenatal vitamin to compensate for your body's increased demand for various vitamins and minerals. Numerous studies have shown that taking a multivitamin up to one month before conception and throughout pregnancy reduces the risk of birth defects.

Be sure to eat enough protein, which provides the building blocks for new cells and tissues. Pregnant women need to eat at least 75 grams of protein daily. Eat lots of fresh vegetables and fruit. These foods are packed with beneficial nutrients and will not add on unwanted pounds. Pregnant women also need to get at least 1,200 milligrams of calcium daily or there is a risk that the baby will leech calcium from your bones, increasing your risk of developing osteoporosis later in life. If your prenatal vitamin doesn't contain enough calcium, ask your doctor whether you should take a supplement. Of course, you should also eat calcium-rich foods.

CURVES TIP · Many pregnant women, particularly those who suffer from nausea or other gastrointestinal problems, find that they do better eating six smaller meals throughout the day than trying to eat three big meals.

EXERCISE · The American College of Obstetricians and Gynecologists (ACOG) recommends that all healthy pregnant women exercise about 30 minutes a day on most days of the week. That sounds right to us! According to the American College of Sports Medicine, pregnant women can reap terrific benefits by maintaining a regular exercise program during pregnancy, including:

- Improved cardiovascular and muscular fitness
- Faster recovery from labor
- Quicker return to prepregnancy weight
- Reduced postpartum belly
- Reduced back pain from pregnancy
- More energy and enhanced feelings of well-being
- Easier pregnancy with fewer obstetric interventions
- Easier labor with shorter active phase of labor and less pain
- Less weight gain during pregnancy, and faster return to post-pregnancy weight

• Increased likelihood of adopting permanent healthy lifestyle habits

CAUTION • Exercise is not for every pregnant woman. Ask your doctor before you embark on an exercise regimen. Women with particular medical problems, such as pregnancy-induced high blood pressure, weak cervix, signs of preterm labor, or slow fetal growth, should not do any strenuous activities.

Not all physical activities are appropriate for pregnant women. If you are allowed to exercise, a daily half-hour walk at a brisk pace is ideal. If you prefer to work out at a gym, the rule of thumb is don't overdo it. Work at a reasonable pace, drink lots of fluids, and dress comfortably with good foot support. Don't work yourself to the point of excess fatigue or exhaustion. Don't lift anything so heavy that it strains your back muscles. The Curves workout should be modified so that you are working at 50 percent of your target heart rate and 50 percent of your strength.

After the fourth month, avoid any activity that strains your waist or forces you to stretch to the point of discomfort.

No scuba diving—it can create gas bubbles in the infant's circulatory system.

WATCH YOUR TUMMY Don't do anything that can risk injury to the abdomen—in other words, kickboxing is out! Needless to say, no contact sports like basketball, ice hockey, or soccer.

DON'T GET OVERHEATED Don't exercise in very hot weather. Stop exercising if you start sweating or feeling warm. Work within your target-heart-rate zone, and don't overdo it. While you are exercising, you should be able to carry on a conversation. You should not be so out of breath that you are huffing and puffing.

WATCH YOUR BALANCE During pregnancy, your joints are more flexible and therefore weaker. This, combined with a larger abdomen, can create balance problems. Particularly after the second trimester, avoid activities that require jogging, jumping, or working on a step.

STAY OFF YOUR BACK After the third month, do not do any exercise lying on your back. The weight of your stomach can cut off the flow of blood to the fetus.

KNOW WHEN TO STOP If you feel sick or faint, experience vaginal bleeding or a rush of fluid from the vagina, abdominal contractions, elevated pulse rate after exercise, chest pain, or decreased fetal movement after exercise, or any other untoward symptom, discontinue exercising and call your doctor.

POSTPARTUM RECOVERY • Most women are able to resume exercise within the six weeks after delivery, but be sure to check with your doctor before embarking on an exercise regimen.

Breast-feeding is not only best for babies—it's a great way to help new mothers take off weight. In fact, a recent study found that women who breast-fed for more than three months after giving birth had the least postpregnancy weight gain. Don't worry, exercising will not interfere with the quality or flow of your breast milk. Some studies suggest that it's best for a new mother to breast-feed before she exercises because the post-workout breast milk may contain more lactic acid, a normal by-product of muscle activity, which may make it less palatable to the infant.

Give your body time to recover. Focus on nutrition and get enough rest (when you can). Make fitness a regular part of your life, and you will not end up as another casualty in the war on obesity.

The Curves Weight-Loss and Fitness Program provides a blueprint to lose weight—permanently and safely—regain your health, and look and feel your best. I've given you the tools to liberate yourself from the tyranny of constant dieting, so that you can eat normally forever.

As good as the Curves program is, it can't work unless you work with it. I would like to share with you some tips on how you can enhance your own results.

CREATE AN ENVIRONMENT FOR SUCCESS · Those of you who truly believe that the Curves program will work for you are already halfway to achieving success. Everything you think and do will reinforce that belief. You'll make sure that your refrigerator is filled with the right food and your head is filled with the right thoughts. You will not allow unsupportive people to thwart your efforts, and you will gravitate to people who are supportive. You will not lose sight of your long-range goal.

If you should slip up, which can happen to even the most motivated people, you will not accept one misstep as failure or as an excuse to quit—you will simply get back on track. You will persevere until you reach your goal.

PICK THE RIGHT GOAL FOR YOU · Creating a successful environment begins with selecting the right goal. First, be sure that your expectations are realistic. Despite the images that you see in fashion magazines, all women are not meant to be superthin or wear a size 4. Real women really do have curves! A woman with a lean, strong, well-toned body can be beautiful in a size 10 or 12, depending on her height and body type. So please don't fixate on the wrong goal for you. If you have a great deal of weight to lose and expect to lose it overnight, you are setting yourself up for disappointment and failure. If you expect too much too soon, you will resort to unhealthy measures that at best are temporary and at worst can lead to permanent damage. Losing a lot of weight can be a daunting task. Celebrate your interim victories. Every day you follow the Curves program, every day you watch your carbohydrate intake or count calories, and every day you do your workout is a day that you can be proud of yourself. Reward yourself every time you drop a dress size or lose five or 10 pounds. Take pride in your accomplishment.

DEVELOP THE HABITS THAT WILL HELP YOU ACHIEVE YOUR GOALS · As I was writing this book, I called Curves centers across the country to check on the progress of our past Sweetheart winners, women who we have recognized for their commitment and excellent results on the Curves program. Some had moved away from Curves or encountered a family crisis that understandably distracted them, at least momentarily, from pursuing their own goals. Among the many women who had kept off the weight, an interesting pattern emerged. These women were very consistent in their exercise habits. When we called their local Curves facility to find them, the fitness manager always knew the day and time that they would be working out. "Oh, Connie's here every afternoon at three," or "Tanya comes every morning at seven-thirty." Exercise has become a habit in these women's lives, and it shows on their bodies.

Similarly, eating healthfully, making the right food choices, and not giving in to destructive impulses can create new lifetime habits. As with any habit, a good habit may take a few weeks or months to take hold, but if you persist, you can replace the bad habits that made you overweight and unhappy with good habits that will give you a lifetime of good health.

MAKE YOURSELF A PRIORITY · Women have a unique place in society. They are expected to be breadwinners, breadmakers, and caregivers of children, husbands, and adult parents. Life is busier than ever. On a positive note, women's lives can be full and fulfilled. On a negative note, too much to do for everyone else can mean too little time for you. I know that time is a precious commodity, and that's why the Curves workout at Curves or at home is only 30 minutes three times a week. Not having enough time to take care of yourself is no excuse! You have to be as diligent about keeping your appointment with yourself as you are about caring for others. You must be serious about your commitment to yourself, whether it's carving out the time to do your workout or going to the store to stock your refrigerator with the right food. It may take some adjustment on the part of family members, but your needs are no less important than theirs. If you take your commitment to yourself seriously, the people who love you and rely on you will support your efforts.

As our nation gets fatter and sicker, it is critical that we reconsider the models of nutrition, weight loss, and health care. A recent survey showed that people blame themselves for obesity and poor health habits, which is only partially true. I believe that much of the responsibility for the poor health of Americans must be borne by health-care professionals who have provided their patients with little or no useful information on nutrition and who have perpetuated the myth that you must diet forever to stay slim. The old paradigm of simply cutting fat and calories to lose weight has produced a 95 percent failure rate. With the help of our 20,000 fitness instructors, including franchisees and their employees, the Curves Weight-Loss and Fitness Program offers a new paradigm of weight loss and health in America.

With Curves, you can enjoy permanent weight loss without permanent dieting, while protecting yourself against many chronic diseases. You are now embarking on an exciting new phase of your life, in which you will wake up every day looking better, and feeling stronger and healthier. Enjoy the journey.

May God bless you with peace, joy, and abundance. See you at Curves!

Gary Heavin
April 2003

PART FOUR

Your

Fitness Planner

Success One Day at a Time

THE CURVES DAILY PLANNER

Carbohydrate-Sensitive Food Plan Shopping Lists

Calorie-Sensitive Food Plan Shopping Lists

Recipes

Multivitamin/Mineral Supplement Shopping List

Daily Meal Planner

Phase 3: Retraining Your Metabolism Chart

The Metabolic Tune-Up Tracking Chart

Weekly Progress Report

CARBOHYDRATE-SENSITIVE FOOD PLAN SHOPPING LISTS

Phase 1 • Week 1

DAIRY

3 tablespoons butter

2 ounces cheddar cheese

2½ cups cottage cheese, 1% fat

9 eggs

3 ounces Havarti cheese

½ gallon skim milk (for protein shakes)

2 tablespoons vegetable cream cheese

8 ounces yogurt, plain

FRUITS

1½ cups cantaloupe, cubed

½ cup strawberries

MEAT

4 strips bacon

10 ounces chicken breast, divided into one 4-ounce and one 6-ounce portion

8-ounce cod fillet

8 ounces cooked salad shrimp

10 ounces ground beef, 93% lean, divided into one 4-ounce and one 6-ounce portion

9 ounces ham, lean, divided into three 3-ounce portions

8 ounces orange roughy

6-ounce pork chop, lean

6 ounces salmon fillet

8 sausage links

6 ounces sirloin steak

2.8-ounce can tuna, in water

4 ounces turkey bacon

4 ounces turkey breast, deli

OTHER

2 dill pickles

2 tablespoons olive oil

RECIPES

(If you are making any of these recipes, please add the ingredients to your shopping list.)

1 serving Chicken Fajitas

1 serving French Onion Soup

1 serving Parmesan Vegetable Stir-Fry

1 serving Tuna Salad

SALAD

7 Free Foods Salads

SHAKES

7 Curves Shakes or other protein shakes

VEGETABLES

1 cup asparagus

½ cup baby carrots

½ cup broccoli florets

½ cup brussels sprouts

1 cup cauliflower florets

4 stalks celery

1 cup spinach

½ cup zucchini

Phase 1 • Week 2

DAIRY

3 tablespoons butter

2 ounces cheddar cheese

3 cups cottage cheese, 1% fat

9 eggs

½ gallon skim milk (for protein shakes)

3 ounces Havarti cheese

2 tablespoons vegetable cream cheese

8 ounces yogurt, plain

FRUITS

1½ cups cantaloupe, cubed

½ cup strawberries

MEAT

4 strips bacon

12 ounces chicken breast, divided into two 6-ounce portions

8-ounce cod fillet

8 ounces cooked salad shrimp

12 ounces ground beef, 93% lean, divided into two 6-ounce portions

9 ounces ham, lean, divided into three 3-ounce portions

8 ounces orange roughy

6 ounces pork chop, lean

4 ounces roast beef, deli

6 ounces salmon fillet

8 sausage links

6 ounces sirloin steak, broiled

2.8-ounce can tuna, in water

4 ounces turkey bacon

4 ounces turkey breast, deli

OTHER

2 dill pickles

2 tablespoons olive oil

RECIPES

(If you are making any of these recipes, please add the ingredients to your shopping list.)

    1 serving Chicken Fajitas

    1 serving French Onion Soup

    1 serving Parmesan Vegetable Stir-Fry

    1 serving Tuna Salad

SALAD

    7 Free Foods Salads

SHAKES

    7 Curves Shakes or other protein shakes

VEGETABLES

    1 cup asparagus

    ½ cup baby carrots

    ½ cup broccoli florets

    ½ cup brussels sprouts

    1 cup cauliflower florets

    4 stalks celery

    1 cup spinach

    ½ cup zucchini

Phase 2 • Week 1

DAIRY

    2 tablespoons butter

    2 ounces cheddar cheese

    1½ cups cottage cheese, 1% fat

    6 eggs

    4 ounces Havarti cheese

    ½ gallon skim milk (for protein shakes)

    2 tablespoons vegetable cream cheese

    12 ounces yogurt, plain

FRUITS

1 apple, small

½ banana

¼ cup blueberries

1 cup cantaloupe, cubed

1 peach, medium

2 plums, medium

1 cup strawberries

MEAT

14 ounces chicken breast, divided into one 8-ounce and one 6-ounce portion

6 ounces chopped sirloin

1 Cornish hen

6 ounces ground beef, 93% lean

8 ounces ham, lean, divided into two 3-ounce and one 2-ounce portion

8 ounces pork chop, lean

4.25-ounce can sardines

8 sausage links

8 ounces scallops

16 ounces shrimp

OTHER

2 ounces almonds, roasted and salted

¼ cup olive oil

½ cup refried beans

4 ounces V8 juice

RECIPES

(If you are making any of these recipes, please add the ingredients to your shopping list.)

1 serving Beef Tenderloin with Blue Cheese

1 serving Buffalo Meatballs

1 serving Chicken Fajitas

1 serving Chinese Vegetables

1 serving French Onion Soup

2 servings Italian Soda

1 serving Lemony Cauliflower

Seafood Marinade

1 serving Spicy Zucchini Boats

1 serving Spinach Salad

1 serving Tofu Stir-Fry

2 servings Tuna Salad

2 servings Vegetable Soup

SALAD

5 Free Foods Salads

SHAKES

7 Curves Shakes or other protein shakes

STARCHES

1 slice bread, whole-wheat

4 Keebler Harvest Bakery Multigrain Crackers

1 piece Holland rusk dry toast

4 RyKrisp crackers

VEGETABLES

½ cup asparagus

2 cups broccoli florets

½ cup mushrooms

½ cup onion

½ cup snow peas

1 cup spinach

1 tomato

2 cups zucchini

Phase 2 • Week 2

DAIRY

5 tablespoons butter

3 ounces cheddar cheese

1½ cups cottage cheese, 1% fat

6 eggs

5 ounces Havarti cheese

1 tablespoon Parmesan cheese, grated

½ gallon skim milk (for protein shakes)

2 tablespoons vegetable cream cheese

8 ounces yogurt, plain

FRUITS

½ banana

¼ cup blueberries

1 cup cantaloupe, cubed

1 orange, medium

1 cup strawberries

½ cup watermelon, cubed

MEAT

14 ounces chicken breast, divided into one 8-ounce and one 6-ounce portion

6-ounce flank steak

12 ounces ground beef, 93% lean, divided into two 6-ounce portions

6 ounces ham, lean, divided into two 3-ounce portions

6-ounce lamb chop

6-ounce pork chop, lean

2 ounces roast beef, deli

9 sausage links

8 ounces shrimp

6 ounces smoked sausage, low-fat

8 ounces trout

OTHER

2 ounces cashews, roasted and salted

1 ounce macadamia nuts

2 tablespoons olive oil

½ cup refried beans

2 tablespoons salsa

½ cup sauerkraut

8 ounces V8 juice

4 ounces wine, rosé

RECIPES

(If you are making any of these recipes, please add the ingredients to your shopping list.)

1 serving Buffalo Meatballs

1 serving Chinese Vegetables

1 serving Easy Frittata

1 serving French Onion Soup

1 serving Greek Salad

1 serving Sherry-Mushroom Chicken

1 serving Spinach Salad with Orange Vinaigrette

1 serving Tofu Stir-Fry

1 serving Tuna Salad

1 serving Vegetable Soup

SALAD

5 Free Foods Salads

SHAKES

7 Curves Shakes or other protein shakes

STARCHES

2 slices bread, whole-wheat

4 Keebler Harvest Bakery Multigrain Crackers

1 piece Holland rusk dry toast

VEGETABLES

½ cup asparagus
½ cup brussels sprouts
1 cup carrots
1 cup cauliflower florets
1 cup green beans
½ cup peas, green
1 cup spinach
1 cup zucchini

Phase 2 • Week 3

DAIRY

2 tablespoons butter
2 ounces cheddar cheese
2 cups cottage cheese, 1% fat
8 eggs
5 ounces Havarti cheese
½ gallon skim milk (for protein shakes)
2 tablespoons vegetable cream cheese
8 ounces yogurt, plain

FRUITS

1 apple, small
¼ cup blueberries
1½ cups cantaloupe, cubed
1 orange, medium
½ cup strawberries
½ cup watermelon, cubed

MEAT

4 slices bacon
14 ounces chicken breast, divided into one 8-ounce and one 6-ounce
portion

6 ounces ground beef, 93% lean

6 ounces halibut

8 ounces ham, lean, divided into two 3-ounce and one 2-ounce portion

8 ounces orange roughy

6-ounce pork chop, lean

4 ounces roast beef, deli

9 sausage links

8 ounces scallops

6 ounces smoked sausage, low-fat

OTHER

1 tablespoon barbeque sauce

2 ounces cashews, roasted and salted

1 tablespoon light mayonnaise

2 tablespoons olive oil

2 ounces pistachio nuts, in shells

½ cup refried beans

½ cup sauerkraut

4 ounces V8 juice

4 ounces wine, rosé

RECIPES

1 serving Beef & Vegetable Stew

1 serving Chicken Fajitas

1 serving Creamy Coleslaw

1 serving Easy Frittata

1 serving Greek Salad

1 serving Italian Soda

1 serving Lemony Cauliflower

1 serving Parmesan Vegetable Stir-Fry

1 serving Sherry-Mushroom Chicken

1 serving Tuna Salad

2 Turkey-Lettuce Wraps

1 serving Vegetable Soup

SALAD

6 Free Foods Salads

SHAKES

7 Curves Shakes or other protein shakes

STARCHES

2 slices bread, whole-wheat

1 piece Keebler Harvest Bakery Multigrain Crackers

1 piece Holland rusk dry toast

2 RyKrisp crackers

VEGETABLES

½ cup asparagus

1 cup broccoli florets

1 cup carrots

1 cup green beans

1 cup mushrooms

½ cup snow peas

1 cup spinach

1 cup zucchini

Phase 2 • Week 4

DAIRY

1 tablespoon blue cheese

4 tablespoons butter

6 ounces cheddar cheese

2 cups cottage cheese, 1% fat

8 eggs

5 ounces Monterey Jack cheese

1 tablespoon Parmesan cheese, grated

½ gallon skim milk (for protein shakes)

2 tablespoons vegetable cream cheese

4 ounces yogurt, plain

FRUITS

¼ cup blueberries

1½ cups cantaloupe, cubed

1 orange, medium

1 plum, medium

1 cup strawberries

1 cup watermelon, cubed

MEAT

4 strips bacon

12 ounces chicken breast, divided into two 6-ounce portions

12 ounces ground beef, 93% lean, divided into two 6-ounce portions

12 ounces ham, lean, divided into four 3-ounce portions

8 ounces orange roughy

6-ounce pork chop, lean

6-ounce salmon fillet

6 sausage links

8-ounce tuna steak (fresh)

OTHER

3 tablespoons olive oil

2 ounces peanuts, dry-roasted

½ cup refried beans

2 tablespoons salsa

½ cup sauerkraut

8 ounces V8 juice

8 ounces wine, rosé

RECIPES

(If you are making any of these recipes, please add the ingredients to your shopping list.)

1 serving Beef & Vegetable Stew

1 serving Beef Tenderloin with Blue Cheese

1 serving French Onion Soup

1 serving Frozen Chocolate Mousse

1 serving Greek Salad

1 serving Italian Soda

1 serving Italian Stuffed Mushrooms

1 serving Jamaican Seafood Medley

Seafood Marinade

1 serving Spicy Chili Pork Chops

1 serving Spicy Zucchini Boats

2 Turkey-Lettuce Wraps

SALADS

6 Free Foods Salads

SHAKES

7 Curves Shakes or other protein shakes

STARCHES

1 slice bread, whole-wheat

4 Keebler Harvest Bakery Multigrain Crackers

1 piece Holland rusk dry toast

4 RyKrisp crackers

VEGETABLES

1 cup asparagus

1 cup broccoli florets

1 cup carrots

1 cup cauliflower florets

¼ cup corn, whole-kernel

1 cup mushrooms

½ cup red bell pepper

½ cup snow peas

1 cup spinach

1½ cups zucchini

Phase 2 • Week 5

DAIRY

> 1 tablespoon blue cheese
>
> 3 tablespoons butter
>
> 4 ounces cheddar cheese
>
> 2 cups cottage cheese, 1% fat
>
> 7 eggs
>
> ½ gallon skim milk (for protein shakes)
>
> 4 ounces Swiss cheese
>
> 2 tablespoons vegetable cream cheese
>
> 4 ounces yogurt, plain

FRUITS

> ½ cup grapes, seedless
>
> 1½ cups strawberries
>
> 1½ cups watermelon, cubed

MEAT

> 8 strips bacon
>
> 18 ounces chicken breast, divided into three 6-ounce portions
>
> 18 ounces ground beef, 93% lean, divided into three 6-ounce portions
>
> 3 ounces ham, lean
>
> 8-ounce pork chop, lean
>
> 8 ounces red snapper
>
> 2 ounces roast beef, deli
>
> 6 sausage links
>
> 8 ounces shrimp
>
> 6-ounce sirloin steak
>
> 8 ounces smoked sausage, low-fat
>
> 2 ounces turkey breast, deli

OTHER

> 1 ounce almonds, roasted and salted
>
> 1 tablespoon barbeque sauce

½ cup French vanilla ice cream

1 tablespoon light mayonnaise

1 ounce macadamia nuts

2 tablespoons olive oil

1 ounce peanuts, dry-roasted

½ cup refried beans

2 tablespoons salsa

½ cup sauerkraut

4 ounces wine, rosé

RECIPES

1 serving Chinese Vegetables

1 serving Creamy Coleslaw

1 serving French Onion Soup

1 serving Frozen Chocolate Mousse

1 serving Italian Stuffed Mushrooms

1 serving Jamaican Seafood Medley

1 serving Lemony Cauliflower

1 serving Sherry-Mushroom Chicken

1 serving Spicy Chili Pork Chops

1 serving Spicy Zucchini Boats

1 serving Spinach Salad with Orange Vinaigrette

1 serving Vegetable Soup

SALAD

6 Free Foods Salads

SHAKES

7 Curves Shakes or other protein shakes

STARCHES

3 slices bread, whole-wheat

4 Keebler Harvest Bakery Multigrain Crackers

1 piece Holland rusk dry toast

VEGETABLES

½ cup baby carrots

1 cup broccoli florets

1 cup green beans

½ cup peas, green

½ cup snow peas

1 cup zucchini

CALORIE-SENSITIVE FOOD PLAN SHOPPING LISTS

Phase 1 • Week 1

DAIRY

> 3 tablespoons butter
>
> 2 ounces cheddar cheese
>
> 2½ cups cottage cheese, 1% fat
>
> 2 eggs
>
> 2 ounces Havarti cheese
>
> ½ gallon skim milk (for protein shakes)
>
> 2 tablespoons vegetable cream cheese
>
> 8 ounces yogurt, plain

FRUITS

> 1 apple, small
>
> ⅜ cup blueberries
>
> 1½ cups cantaloupe, cubed
>
> 1 grapefruit
>
> 1 orange, medium
>
> ½ cup strawberries

MEAT

> 8-ounce chicken breast, divided into two 4-ounce portions
>
> 8 ounces cod fillet
>
> 8 ounces ground beef, 93% lean, divided into two 4-ounce portions
>
> 9 ounces ham, lean, divided into three 3-ounce portions
>
> 8 ounces orange roughy
>
> 4-ounce pork chop, lean
>
> 4 ounces roast beef, deli
>
> 4-ounce salmon fillet
>
> 7 sausage links
>
> 4-ounce sirloin steak

2.8-ounce can tuna, packed in water

4 ounces turkey breast, deli

OTHER

2 dill pickles

2 tablespoons olive oil

2 ounces peanuts, dry-roasted

8 ounces V8 juice

RECIPES

(If you are making any of these recipes, please add the ingredients to your shopping list.)

1 serving Chicken Fajitas

1 serving French Onion Soup

1 serving Parmesan Vegetable Stir-Fry

1 serving Tuna Salad

1 serving Vegetable Soup

SALAD

7 Free Foods Salads

SHAKES

7 Curves Shakes or other protein shakes

STARCHES

4 slices bread, whole-wheat

2 Keebler Harvest Bakery Multigrain Crackers

4 RyKrisp crackers

VEGETABLES

½ cup baby carrots

½ cup broccoli florets

½ cup brussels sprouts

1 cup cauliflower florets

2 celery stalks

½ cup peas, green
1 cup spinach
1 tomato
½ cup zucchini

Phase 1 • Week 2

DAIRY

3 tablespoons butter
2 ounces cheddar cheese
2½ cups cottage cheese
2 eggs
½ gallon skim milk (for protein shakes)
2 ounces Havarti cheese
2 tablespoons vegetable cream cheese
8 ounces yogurt, plain

FRUITS

1 apple, small
⅜ cup blueberries
1½ cups cantaloupe, cubed
1 grapefruit
1 orange, medium
½ cup strawberries

MEAT

8 ounces chicken breast, divided into two 4-ounce portions
8 ounces cod fillet
8 ounces ground beef, 93% lean, divided into two 4-ounce portions
9 ounces ham, lean, divided into three 3-ounce portions
8 ounces orange roughy
4-ounce pork chop, lean
4 ounces roast beef, deli
4-ounce salmon fillet

8 sausage links

4-ounce sirloin steak, broiled

2.8-ounce can tuna, in water

4 ounces turkey breast, deli

OTHER

2 dill pickles

2 tablespoons olive oil

2 ounces peanuts, dry-roasted

8 ounces V8 juice

RECIPES

(If you are making any of these recipes, please add the ingredients to your shopping list.)

1 serving Chicken Fajitas

1 serving French Onion Soup

1 serving Parmesan Vegetable Stir-Fry

1 serving Tuna Salad

1 serving Vegetable Soup

SALAD

7 Free Foods Salads

SHAKES

7 Curves Shakes or other protein shakes

STARCHES

4 slices bread, whole-wheat

2 Keebler Harvest Bakery Multigrain Crackers

4 RyKrisp crackers

VEGETABLES

½ cup baby carrots

½ cup broccoli florets

½ cup brussels sprouts

1 cup cauliflower florets

2 celery stalks

½ cup peas, green

1 cup spinach

1 tomato

½ cup zucchini

Phase 2 • Week 1

DAIRY

2 tablespoons butter

1 ounce cheddar cheese

1½ cups cottage cheese, 1% fat

5 eggs

4 ounces Havarti cheese

½ gallon skim milk (for protein shakes)

4 tablespoons vegetable cream cheese

20 ounces yogurt, plain

FRUITS

1 apple, small

½ banana

¼ cup blueberries

1 cup cantaloupe, cubed

1 orange, medium

1 peach, medium

1 cup strawberries

MEAT

14 ounces chicken breast, divided into one 8-ounce and one 6-ounce
portion

6 ounces chopped sirloin

1 Cornish hen

4 ounces ground beef, 93% lean

8 ounces ham, lean, divided into two 3-ounce and one 2-ounce portion

8-ounce pork chop, lean

4.25-ounce can sardines

7 sausage links

8 ounces scallops

16 ounces shrimp

OTHER

2 ounces almonds, roasted and salted

¼ cup olive oil

½ cup refried beans

20 ounces V8 juice

RECIPES

(If you are making any of these recipes, please add the ingredients to your shopping list.)

1 serving Beef Tenderloin with Blue Cheese

1 serving Buffalo Meatballs

1 serving Chicken Fajitas

1 serving Chinese Vegetables

1 serving French Onion Soup

1 serving Italian Soda

1 serving Lemony Cauliflower

Seafood Marinade

2 servings Spicy Zucchini Boats

1 serving Spinach Salad with Orange Vinaigrette

1 serving Tofu Stir-Fry

2 servings Tuna Salad

1 serving Vegetable Soup

SALAD

5 Free Foods Salads

SHAKES

7 Curves Shakes or other protein shakes

STARCHES

2 slices bread, whole-wheat

4 Keebler Harvest Bakery Multigrain Crackers

4 RyKrisp crackers

VEGETABLES

3 artichoke heart pieces

½ cup asparagus

2 cups broccoli florets

½ cup mushrooms

½ cup onion

1 cup spinach

1 tomato

2 cups zucchini

Phase 2 • Week 2

DAIRY

3 tablespoons butter

3 ounces cheddar cheese

1½ cups cottage cheese, 1% fat

6 eggs

4 ounces Havarti cheese

1 tablespoon Parmesan cheese, grated

½ gallon skim milk (for protein shakes)

2 tablespoons vegetable cream cheese

8 ounces yogurt, plain

FRUITS

1 apple, small

½ banana

¼ cup blueberries

1 cup cantaloupe, cubed

1 orange, medium

1 cup strawberries

½ cup watermelon, cubed

MEAT

4 strips bacon

14 ounces chicken breast, divided into one 8-ounce and one 6-ounce
portion

6-ounce flank steak

10 ounces ground beef, 93% lean, divided into one 6-ounce and one
4-ounce portion

6-ounces ham, lean, divided into two 3-ounce portions

4-ounce lamb chop

4-ounce pork chop, lean

2 ounces roast beef, deli

5 sausage links

8 ounces shrimp

6 ounces smoked sausage, low-fat

6 ounces trout

OTHER

2 ounces cashews, roasted and salted

1 tablespoon light mayonnaise

1 ounce macadamia nuts

2 tablespoons olive oil

½ cup refried beans

2 tablespoons salsa

½ cup sauerkraut

20 ounces V8 juice

4 ounces wine, rosé

RECIPES

*(If you are making any of these recipes, please add the ingredients to
your shopping list.)*

1 serving Buffalo Meatballs

1 serving Chinese Vegetables

1 serving Easy Frittata

1 serving French Onion Soup

1 serving Greek Salad

1 serving Sherry-Mushroom Chicken

1 serving Spinach Salad with Orange Vinaigrette

1 serving Tofu Stir-Fry

1 serving Tuna Salad

1 serving Vegetable Soup

SALAD

5 Free Foods Salads

SHAKES

7 Curves Shakes or other protein shakes

STARCHES

2 slices bread, whole-wheat

4 Keebler Harvest Bakery Multigrain Crackers

2 pieces Holland rusk dry toast

VEGETABLES

½ cup asparagus

½ cup brussels sprouts

1 cup carrots

1 cup cauliflower florets

1 cup green beans

½ cup peas, green

1 cup spinach

½ tomato

1 cup zucchini

Phase 2 · Week 3

DAIRY

2 tablespoons butter

1 ounce cheddar cheese

2 cups cottage cheese, 1% fat

8 eggs

5 ounces Havarti cheese

½ gallon skim milk (for protein shakes)

2 tablespoons vegetable cream cheese

8 ounces yogurt, plain

FRUITS

1 apple, small

¼ cup blueberries

1½ cups cantaloupe, cubed

1 orange, medium

½ cup strawberries

½ cup watermelon, cubed

MEAT

4 strips bacon

14 ounces chicken breast, divided into one 8-ounce and one 6-ounce
portion

6 ounces ground beef, 93% lean

5 ounces halibut

8 ounces ham, lean, divided into two 3-ounce and one 2-ounce
portion

8 ounces orange roughy

6-ounce pork chop, lean

4 ounces roast beef, deli

9 sausage links

8 ounces scallops

6 ounces smoked sausage, light

OTHER

> 1 tablespoon barbeque sauce
>
> 3 ounces cashews, roasted and salted
>
> 1 tablespoon light mayonnaise
>
> 2 tablespoons olive oil
>
> 2 ounces pistachio nuts, in shells
>
> ½ cup refried beans
>
> ½ cup sauerkraut
>
> 8 ounces V8 juice
>
> 4 ounces wine, rosé

RECIPES

> *(If you are making any of these recipes, please add the ingredients to your shopping list.)*
>
> 1 serving Beef & Vegetable Stew
>
> 1 serving Chicken Fajitas
>
> 1 serving Creamy Coleslaw
>
> 1 serving Easy Frittata
>
> 1 serving Greek Salad
>
> 1 serving Italian Soda
>
> 1 serving Lemony Cauliflower
>
> 1 serving Parmesan Vegetable Stir-Fry
>
> 1 serving Sherry-Mushroom Chicken
>
> 1 serving Tuna Salad
>
> 2 Turkey-Lettuce Wraps
>
> 1 serving Vegetable Soup

SALAD

> 6 Free Foods Salads

SHAKES

> 7 Curves Shakes or other protein shakes

STARCHES

> 2 slices bread, whole-wheat

2 Keebler Harvest Bakery Multigrain Crackers

2 pieces Holland rusk dry toast

2 RyKrisp crackers

VEGETABLES

½ cup asparagus

1 cup broccoli florets

1 cup carrots

1 cup green beans

1 cup mushrooms

½ cup snow peas

1 cup spinach

1 cup zucchini

Phase 2 • Week 4

DAIRY

3 tablespoons butter

6 ounces cheddar cheese

2 cups cottage cheese, 1% fat

7 eggs

5 ounces Monterey Jack cheese

1 tablespoon Parmesan cheese, grated

½ gallon skim milk (for protein shakes)

2 tablespoons vegetable cream cheese

8 ounces yogurt, plain

FRUITS

1 apple, small

¼ cup blueberries

1½ cups cantaloupe, cubed

1 plum, medium

1 cup strawberries

1 cup watermelon, cubed

MEAT

4 strips bacon

12 ounces chicken breast, divided into two 6-ounce portions

10 ounces ground beef, 93% lean, divided into one 6-ounce and one
4-ounce portion

11 ounces ham, lean, divided into three 3-ounce and one 2-ounce
portion

8 ounces orange roughy

6-ounce pork chop, lean

4-ounce salmon fillet

6 sausage links

8-ounce tuna steak (fresh)

OTHER

3 tablespoons olive oil

2 ounces peanuts, dry-roasted

½ cup refried beans

2 tablespoons salsa

½ cup sauerkraut

8 ounces V8 juice

8 ounces wine, rosé

RECIPES

*(If you are making any of these recipes, please add the ingredients to
your shopping list.)*

1 serving Beef & Vegetable Stew

1 serving Beef Tenderloin with Blue Cheese

1 serving French Onion Soup

1 serving Frozen Chocolate Mousse

1 serving Greek Salad

1 serving Italian Soda

1 serving Italian Stuffed Mushrooms

1 serving Jamaican Seafood Medley

Seafood Marinade

1 serving Spicy Chili Pork Chops

1 serving Spicy Zucchini Boats

2 Turkey-Lettuce Wraps

SALAD

6 Free Foods Salads

SHAKES

7 Curves Shakes or other protein shakes

STARCHES

1 slice bread, whole-wheat

4 Keebler Harvest Bakery Multigrain Crackers

1 piece Holland rusk dry toast

4 RyKrisp crackers

VEGETABLES

1 cup asparagus

1 cup broccoli florets

1 cup carrots

1 cup cauliflower florets

½ cup corn, whole-kernel

1 cup mushrooms

½ cup red bell pepper

½ cup snow peas

1 cup spinach

1½ cups zucchini

Phase 2 • Week 5

DAIRY

3 tablespoons butter

1 tablespoon blue cheese

4 ounces cheddar cheese

2 cups cottage cheese, 1% fat

7 eggs

½ gallon skim milk (for protein shakes)

3 ounces Swiss cheese

2 tablespoons vegetable cream cheese

4 ounces yogurt, plain

FRUITS

½ cup grapes, seedless

1 peach, medium

1½ cups strawberries

1½ cups watermelon, cubed

MEAT

8 strips bacon

18 ounces chicken breast, divided into three 6-ounce portions

16 ounces ground beef, 93% lean, divided into two 6-ounce and one
4-ounce portion

2 ounces ham, lean

8-ounce pork chop, lean

8 ounces red snapper

2 ounces roast beef, deli

6 sausage links

8 ounces shrimp

6-ounce sirloin steak, broiled

8 ounces smoked sausage, low-fat

2 ounces turkey breast, deli

OTHER

1 ounce almonds, roasted and salted

1 tablespoon barbeque sauce

½ cup French vanilla ice cream

1 tablespoon light mayonnaise

1 ounce macadamia nuts

2 tablespoons olive oil

1 ounce peanuts, dry-roasted

½ cup refried beans

2 tablespoons salsa

½ cup sauerkraut

4 ounces wine, rosé

RECIPES

(If you are making any of these recipes, please add the ingredients to your shopping list.)

1 serving Chinese Vegetables

1 serving Creamy Coleslaw

1 serving French Onion Soup

1 serving Frozen Chocolate Mousse

1 serving Italian Stuffed Mushrooms

1 serving Jamaican Seafood Medley

1 serving Lemony Cauliflower

1 serving Sherry-Mushroom Chicken

1 serving Spicy Chili Pork Chops

1 serving Spicy Zucchini Boats

1 serving Spinach Salad with Orange Vinaigrette

1 serving Vegetable Soup

SALAD

6 Free Foods Salads

SHAKES

7 Curves Shakes or other protein shakes

STARCHES

3 slices bread, whole-wheat

4 Keebler Harvest Bakery Multigrain Crackers

1 piece Holland rusk dry toast

VEGETABLES

½ cup baby carrots

1 cup broccoli florets

1 cup green beans

½ cup peas, green

½ cup snow peas

1 cup zucchini

RECIPES

SPINACH SALAD with ORANGE VINAIGRETTE

PREPARATION TIME: *15 minutes*

VINAIGRETTE:

2½ tablespoons orange juice

1 tablespoon wine vinegar

1½ tablespoons olive oil

¼ teaspoon ground black pepper

½ teaspoon salt

SALAD:

2 cups fresh baby spinach (lightly packed)

½ cup sliced mushrooms

½ cup thinly sliced red onion

VINAIGRETTE: Combine orange juice and vinegar in shaker. Add oil, pepper, and salt. Shake well.

SALAD: Place salad ingredients in a serving bowl. Toss with vinaigrette to coat vegetables. Serve immediately.

Makes 2 servings

CURVES DIETERS: 3 carbs, 101 calories (per serving)

Free Foods in this recipe: spinach, mushrooms, and onion

Nutritional Information (per serving): Calories: 138, Fat: 10g, Saturated Fat: 0g, Protein: 2g, Carbohydrates: 11g, Fiber: 2g, Cholesterol: 0mg, Sodium: 577mg

GREEK SALAD

PREPARATION TIME: *20 minutes (not including marinating)*

4 ounces cooked chicken breast (no skin or breading), sliced

DRESSING:

1½ tablespoons olive oil

1½ tablespoons lemon juice

1 clove garlic, mashed

½ teaspoon lemon-pepper seasoning

¼ teaspoon salt

¼ teaspoon dried oregano

¼ teaspoon dried basil

SALAD:

2 cups romaine lettuce or iceberg lettuce (or a mixture)

⅛ cucumber, sliced

½ tomato, chopped

⅛ cup thinly sliced red onion

1 tablespoon sliced black olives

1 tablespoon reduced-fat feta cheese, crumbled

Whisk together dressing ingredients and pour over cooked, sliced chicken breast. Marinate in the refrigerator at least 1 hour. Make salad and toss with chicken and dressing.

Makes 1 serving

CURVES DIETERS: 6 carbs, 348 calories (per serving)

Free Foods in this recipe: lemon juice, garlic, romaine lettuce, cucumber, and onion

Nutritional Information (per serving): Calories: 383, Fat: 24g, Saturated Fat: .5g, Protein: 29g, Carbohydrates: 14g, Fiber: 2g, Cholesterol: 64mg, Sodium: 949mg

CREAMY COLESLAW

PREPARATION TIME: *10 minutes (not including chilling)*

DRESSING:

2 tablespoons heavy cream

2 tablespoons light mayonnaise

1 tablespoon vinegar

½ tablespoon sugar

½ teaspoon salt

½ teaspoon whole celery seed

½ teaspoon ground black pepper

4 cups (packed) shredded cabbage (approximately 8 ounces)

Mix dressing ingredients well. Pour over cabbage, and mix. Chill until cold (at least 1 hour). The mixture will pack down to about 1½ cups.

Makes 3 (½-cup) servings

CURVES DIETERS: 3 carbs, 78 calories (per serving)

Free Foods in this recipe: cabbage

Nutritional Information (per serving): Calories: 99, Fat: 7g, Saturated Fat: 3g, Protein: 0g, Carbohydrates: 8g, Fiber: 1g, Cholesterol: 14mg, Sodium: 449mg

FRENCH ONION SOUP

PREPARATION TIME: *2 hours*

4 tablespoons butter (½ stick)

4 cups thinly sliced onions (2 to 3 onions)

2 cups sliced mushrooms

1½ tablespoons flour

6 cups beef broth (not bouillon)

½ teaspoon salt

½ teaspoon ground black pepper

½ cup brandy

½ teaspoon Kitchen Bouquet seasoning

In a 3-quart soup pot on the stovetop, melt butter and add onions, stirring constantly. Cook for 15 to 20 minutes, or until soft. When onions are soft, add mushrooms and cook 2 more minutes. Sprinkle flour over and stir well. Add 2 cups of beef broth. Continue stirring until the mixture is thickened. Add remaining broth and stir in salt, pepper, and brandy. Bring to a boil. Cover and simmer for 45 minutes. Add Kitchen Bouquet seasoning and stir well. Taste for seasoning, and correct if necessary.

Makes 6 (1⅓-cup) servings

CURVES DIETERS: 3 carbs, 145 calories (per serving)
Free Foods in this recipe: onion and mushrooms
Nutritional Information (per serving): Calories: 199, Fat: 8.5g, Saturated Fat:
6g, Protein: 4g, Carbohydrates: 15g, Fiber: 3g, Cholesterol: 21mg, Sodium:
1,735mg

VEGETABLE SOUP

PREPARATION TIME: *2 hours*

1 onion, diced (about 1½ cups)
2 stalks celery, diced
½ cup diced carrots
1 cup shredded green cabbage
3 tablespoons olive oil
2 cloves garlic, minced
1 cup diced zucchini
1 cup diced mushrooms
4 cups fat-free chicken broth
11.5-ounce can tomato juice
1 tablespoon dried parsley flakes
2 cups chopped fresh spinach,
    lightly packed
½ teaspoon salt
¼ teaspoon ground black pepper
1 tablespoon lemon juice

In 3-quart soup pot, saute onion, celery, carrots, and cabbage in olive
oil for 10 minutes, stirring often. Add garlic, zucchini, and
mushrooms, and saute 10 more minutes, stirring often. Add chicken
broth, tomato juice, and parsley flakes. Bring to a boil. Cover and
simmer for 1 hour. Add spinach, salt, pepper, and lemon juice, and
simmer another 15 minutes. Taste and adjust seasoning.

Makes 6 (1-cup) servings

CURVES DIETERS: 5 carbs, 85 calories (per serving)

Free Foods in this recipe: onion, celery, cabbage, garlic, zucchini, mushrooms, parsley, spinach, and lemon juice

Nutritional Information (per serving): Calories: 117, Fat: 7g, Saturated Fat: 1g, Protein: 2g, Carbohydrates: 12g, Fiber: 2g, Cholesterol: 0mg, Sodium: 759mg

BUFFALO MEATBALLS

PREPARATION TIME: *40 minutes*

1 pound ground buffalo meat

¼ cup shredded carrot

¼ cup shredded zucchini

¼ cup shredded onion

1 tablespoon dried parsley flakes

1 teaspoon ground mustard

¼ teaspoon whole celery seed

½ teaspoon salt

¼ teaspoon ground black pepper

1 egg

1 tablespoon Worcestershire sauce

2 tablespoons heavy cream

Mix meat, shredded vegetables, and seasonings very well. Beat egg, Worcestershire sauce, and cream together and add to meat mixture. Mix very well. Scoop up by rounded tablespoonfuls and form into meatballs. On a lightly greased broiler pan, broil 8 minutes. Turn meatballs and broil another 8 minutes.

Makes 4 (5-meatball) servings

CURVES DIETERS: 2 carbs, 243 calories (per serving)

Free Foods in this recipe: zucchini, onion, and parsley

Nutritional Information (per serving): Calories: 248, Fat: 15g, Saturated Fat: 7.5g, Protein: 25g, Carbohydrates: 4g, Fiber: 0g, Cholesterol: 133mg, Sodium: 429mg

CHICKEN FAJITAS

PREPARATION TIME: *20 minutes*

2 tablespoons olive oil
10 ounces chicken breast (boneless and skinless), sliced
½ onion, julienned (about ¾ cup)
¼ green pepper, julienned
¼ red pepper, julienned
1 teaspoon chili powder
½ teaspoon powdered cumin
1 teaspoon salt
2 tablespoons chopped fresh cilantro

In a large skillet, heat olive oil. Add chicken and onion, and saute for 5 minutes, stirring often. Add peppers, chili powder, cumin, and salt, and cook for 5 minutes, stirring often. Stir in cilantro and serve.

Makes 2 servings

CURVES DIETERS: 1 carb, 280 calories (per serving)
Free Foods in this recipe: onion, peppers, and cilantro
Nutritional Information (per serving): Calories: 308, Fat: 16g, Saturated Fat: 2.5g, Protein: 34g, Carbohydrates: 8g, Fiber: 1g, Cholesterol: 80mg, Sodium: 648mg

TURKEY-LETTUCE WRAPS

PREPARATION TIME: *10 minutes*

8 butter lettuce leaves
½ cup vegetable cream cheese, softened
½ cucumber, peeled and diced
¼ cup roasted and salted sunflower seed kernels
8 (½-ounce) slices deli turkey breast

Spread each lettuce leaf with 1 tablespoon cream cheese. Evenly divide cucumber and sunflower seeds between lettuce leaves, and sprinkle over cream cheese. Top each lettuce leaf with 1 slice of turkey. Press down gently and roll up.

Makes 8 wraps

CURVES DIETERS: 6 carbs, 83 calories (per wrap)

Free Foods in this recipe: lettuce and cucumber

Nutritional Information (per wrap): Calories: 87, Fat: 6g, Saturated Fat: 3g, Protein: 5g, Carbohydrates: 7g, Fiber: 0g, Cholesterol: 20mg, Sodium: 254mg

ITALIAN STUFFED MUSHROOMS

PREPARATION TIME: *30 minutes*

¼ pound bulk Italian sausage

½ cup minced onion

2 cloves garlic, minced

½ cup shredded zucchini

½ teaspoon dried oregano

¼ teaspoon dried thyme

1 teaspoon dried parsley flakes

½ teaspoon salt

3 RyKrisp crackers, smashed into fine crumbs (approximately ¼ cup)

2 tablespoons shredded Parmesan cheese

2 tablespoons red wine

2 tablespoons water

18 large button mushrooms, washed and dried

Spray skillet with cooking spray. Brown sausage, breaking up into small crumbles as it cooks. Add onion and cook until tender. Add garlic, zucchini, and spices, and cook well. Turn off heat under skillet. Add cracker crumbs, cheese, wine, and water, and mix well. Remove and discard stems from mushrooms. Stuff mushroom caps with filling, piling high. Place in a glass dish and cover tightly with microwave-safe plastic wrap. Microwave on high power 6 to 8 minutes. Let stand 5 to 7 minutes before serving.

Makes 3 (6-mushroom) servings

CURVES DIETERS: 13 carbs, 177 calories (per serving)

Free Foods in this recipe: onion, garlic, zucchini, parsley, and mushrooms

Nutritional Information (per serving): Calories: 192, Fat: 9g, Saturated Fat: 3g, Protein: 9g, Carbohydrates: 16g, Fiber: 4g, Cholesterol: 24mg, Sodium: 734mg

TUNA SALAD

PREPARATION TIME: *10 minutes*

1 (6-ounce) can solid white albacore tuna (in water)

1 green onion, minced

½ stalk celery, minced

1 radish, minced

½ teaspoon lemon juice

½ teaspoon lemon-pepper seasoning

½ tablespoon yellow mustard

1½ tablespoons light mayonnaise

Drain tuna and break up with a fork. Add remaining ingredients and mix well.

Makes 1 (⅔-cup) serving

CURVES DIETERS: 3 carbs, 258 calories (per serving)

Free Foods in this recipe: green onion, celery, radish, lemon juice, and yellow mustard

Nutritional Information (per serving): Calories: 264, Fat: 12.5g, Saturated Fat: 3.5g, Protein: 34g, Carbohydrates: 4g, Fiber: 0g, Cholesterol: 75mg, Sodium: 1,309mg

BEEF & VEGETABLE STEW

PREPARATION TIME: *8 hours in Crock-Pot*

2 pounds lean beef stew meat

1 tablespoon olive oil

1 onion, thinly sliced

1 green pepper, julienned

6 stalks celery, thinly sliced

4 cups baby carrots

3 cloves garlic, minced

1 cup V8 juice

1 teaspoon Heinz 57 steak sauce

1 teaspoon Worcestershire sauce

¼ cup red wine

½ cup beef broth

1 teaspoon dried parsley flakes

1 tablespoon cornstarch

1 tablespoon water

Brown beef in olive oil. Place meat and drippings in a large Crock-Pot. Place vegetables and garlic on top of meat. Mix liquid ingredients and parsley and pour into Crock-Pot. Cook on high for 7 hours. One hour before serving, stir cornstarch and water together until smooth. Stir into stew, mix well, and continue cooking. Before serving, taste and adjust seasonings, if necessary.

Makes 8 (1-cup) servings

CURVES DIETERS: 8 carbs, 256 calories (per serving)

Free Foods in this recipe: onion, green pepper, celery, garlic, and parsley

Nutritional Information (per serving): Calories: 280, Fat: 14g, Saturated Fat: 5g, Protein: 24g, Carbohydrates: 13g, Fiber: 3g, Cholesterol: 60mg, Sodium: 251mg

Recipes

BEEF TENDERLOIN with BLUE CHEESE

PREPARATION TIME: *1 hour, 15 minutes*

MARINADE:

1 tablespoon olive oil

¼ cup red wine

1 clove garlic, mashed

1 tablespoon tomato paste

1 tablespoon chopped fresh parsley

½ teaspoon freshly cracked black pepper

6 (6-ounce) pieces beef tenderloin, 1½ to 2 inches thick

3 tablespoons crumbled blue cheese

Mix marinade ingredients in a large baking dish. Coat both sides of meat with the marinade and let sit in the refrigerator for 30 to 45 minutes. Grill tenderloin over medium-high heat, or broil 6 inches from heat source, until cooked to taste. (Medium doneness is recommended—about 160 degrees on a meat thermometer.) Top with blue cheese and cook until cheese melts.

Makes 6 servings

CURVES DIETERS: 1 carb, 383 calories (per serving)

Free Foods in this recipe: garlic and parsley

Nutritional Information (per serving): Calories: 383, Fat: 24g, Saturated Fat: 10g, Protein: 38g, Carbohydrates: 1g, Fiber: 0g, Cholesterol: 120mg, Sodium: 470mg

EASY FRITTATA

PREPARATION TIME: *15 minutes*

½ pound ground beef, 93% lean

1 tablespoon butter

2 cups sliced mushrooms

½ onion, chopped (approximately ¾ cup)

2 teaspoons Worcestershire sauce

1 teaspoon ground oregano

½ teaspoon garlic powder

1 teaspoon salt

¼ teaspoon ground black pepper

1 teaspoon dried parsley flakes

2 cups chopped fresh spinach (lightly packed)

4 large eggs

¼ cup skim milk

½ cup shredded Parmesan cheese

Spray a large skillet with cooking spray. Add ground beef, butter, mushrooms, and onion. Cook over medium-high heat 6 to 8 minutes, breaking beef apart with spoon. Add Worcestershire sauce and seasonings. Cook until meat is no longer pink and onion is tender. Stir spinach into meat mixture. Push mixture to one side of skillet. Reduce heat to medium. Beat eggs with skim milk and pour into empty side of the skillet. Cook without stirring for 2 minutes, or until set on the bottom. Lift eggs to allow uncooked portion to flow underneath. Repeat until softly set. Gently stir into meat mixture. Stir in cheese and heat through.

Makes 3 servings

CURVES DIETERS: 4 carbs, 325 calories (per serving)

Free Foods in this recipe: mushrooms, onion, parsley, and spinach

Nutritional Information (per serving): Calories: 384, Fat: 21g, Saturated Fat: 10g, Protein: 33g, Carbohydrates: 16g, Fiber: 4g, Cholesterol: 356mg, Sodium: 1,176mg

JAMAICAN SEAFOOD MEDLEY

PREPARATION TIME: *45 minutes (not counting marinating)*

MARINADE:

2 tablespoons packed brown sugar

1½ tablespoons orange juice

1½ tablespoons lime juice

2 cloves garlic, minced

½ teaspoon ginger, minced

1 teaspoon orange peel, grated

1 teaspoon lime peel, grated

1 teaspoon salt

½ teaspoon ground black pepper

⅛ teaspoon ground cinnamon

dash ground cloves

½ teaspoon Tabasco sauce

½ pound orange roughy, cut into bite-size pieces

½ pound sea scallops, cut in half (or quarters, if very large)

½ pound shrimp, shelled and deveined

1 tablespoon olive oil

¾ cup baby corn, snapped in fourths

1 tablespoon sliced green onion

½ green pepper, julienned

Combine marinade ingredients. Pour over seafood and mix well. Cover and refrigerate at least 2 hours. Drain seafood and discard marinade. Saute seafood and vegetables in olive oil over medium heat for 15 minutes or until done.

Makes 3 servings

CURVES DIETERS: 6 carbs, 283 calories (per serving)

Free Foods in this recipe: garlic, green onion, and green pepper

Nutritional Information (per serving): Calories: 287, Fat: 10.5g, Saturated Fat: .5g, Protein: 41g, Carbohydrates: 7g, Fiber: 2g, Cholesterol: 156mg, Sodium: 433mg

TOFU STIR-FRY

PREPARATION TIME: *15 minutes (not counting preparing tofu for use)*

3 ounces firm tofu (⅕ block)
2 tablespoons olive oil
½ onion, thinly sliced (approximately ¾ cup)
1 clove garlic, minced
½ cup sliced mushrooms
½ cup sliced zucchini
½ cup fresh spinach (packed)
1 tablespoon soy sauce
1 tablespoon water

Press water from tofu by putting it between several layers of paper towels and placing a dinner plate on top. Let sit 20 to 30 minutes. Divide block into 5 portions. (Unused tofu portions may be frozen in individual bags for later use.)

Cube 1 portion tofu and stir-fry in olive oil. Add onion and garlic and cook 4 minutes. Add mushrooms and cook until soft. Add zucchini and cook a few more minutes. Add spinach, soy sauce, and water. Stir well and cook 2 more minutes.

Makes 1 serving

CURVES DIETERS: 2 carbs, 340 calories (per serving)
Free Foods in this recipe: onion, garlic, mushrooms, zucchini, and spinach
Nutritional Information (per serving): Calories: 440, Fat: 31.5g, Saturated Fat: 1g, Protein: 12g, Carbohydrates: 25g, Fiber: 4g, Cholesterol: 0mg, Sodium: 989mg

SEAFOOD MARINADE

PREPARATION TIME: *5 minutes*

    2 tablespoons olive oil

    2 tablespoons seasoned rice vinegar

    1 tablespoon balsamic vinegar

    1 tablespoon lime juice

    1 teaspoon dried chives (or 1 tablespoon fresh chives)

    1 teaspoon dried dill weed (or 1 tablespoon fresh dill)

    1 teaspoon lemon-pepper seasoning

Mix well. Marinate 1 pound of any seafood or fish at least 4 hours. Drain well and discard marinade. Grill or broil seafood until done.

CURVES DIETERS: 2 carbs, 30 calories (per 8 ounces of marinated seafood)
Free Foods in this recipe: none
Nutritional Information (approximately 20% of the marinade will remain with the food and add the following): Calories: 59, Fat: 5.5g, Saturated Fat: 1g, Protein: 0g, Carbohydrates: 3g, Fiber: 0g, Cholesterol: 0mg, Sodium: 201mg

SHERRY-MUSHROOM CHICKEN

PREPARATION TIME: *45 minutes*

    2 tablespoons olive oil

    3 (6-ounce) boneless, skinless chicken breasts

    1½ cups chopped fresh mushrooms

    2 tablespoons sliced green onion

    1 clove garlic, minced

    1 tablespoon cornstarch

    1 tablespoon chopped fresh parsley

    ½ teaspoon dried thyme

    dash ground black pepper

⅔ cup chicken broth
1 tablespoon dry sherry

In a large skillet, saute chicken breasts in olive oil for 15 minutes, or until done on both sides. When cooked, remove and keep warm in the oven while you prepare the sauce. Saute mushrooms, green onion, and garlic in skillet over medium heat until tender. Stir in cornstarch, parsley, thyme, and pepper. Stir in broth and sherry. Cook and stir until sauce boils and thickens. Serve sauce over chicken.

Makes 3 servings

CURVES DIETERS: 3 carbs, 288 calories (per serving)
Free Foods in this recipe: mushrooms, green onion, garlic, and parsley
Nutritional Information (per serving): Calories: 314, Fat: 11.5g, Saturated Fat: 1g, Protein: 43g, Carbohydrates: 8g, Fiber: 1g, Cholesterol: 96mg, Sodium: 113mg

SPICY CHILI PORK CHOPS

PREPARATION TIME: *25 minutes*

4 boneless pork chops (4 ounces each)

RUB:

½ tablespoon salt
½ tablespoon powdered cumin
½ tablespoon ground black pepper
½ tablespoon chili powder
1 tablespoon paprika
½ tablespoon garlic powder
½ tablespoon ground ginger

Trim fat from pork chops. Mix spices together. Rub spice mixture into all sides of meat. Broil or grill 10 to 15 minutes on each side or until done to taste.

Makes 4 servings

CURVES DIETERS: 4 carbs, 219 calories (per serving)
Free Foods in this recipe: none
Nutritional Information (per serving): Calories: 219, Fat: 14g, Saturated Fat: 2.5g, Protein: 19g, Carbohydrates: 4g, Fiber: 0g, Cholesterol: 2mg, Sodium: 1,652mg

CHINESE VEGETABLES

PREPARATION TIME: *30 minutes*

2 tablespoons olive oil
1 tablespoon sesame oil
2 stalks celery, julienned
½ onion, thinly sliced (about ¾ cup)
2 medium carrots, peeled and julienned
¼ cup bamboo shoots, drained well
¼ cup bean sprouts, drained well
½ cup thinly sliced purple cabbage
½ cup snow peas, cut in half
½ cup sliced mushrooms
2 cloves garlic, minced
½ cup chicken broth
1 tablespoon soy sauce
1 tablespoon cornstarch

Heat olive and sesame oils in a large skillet. Add vegetables and saute for 15 minutes, stirring often. Stir chicken broth, soy sauce, and cornstarch together until smooth. Add to skillet and cook until sauce boils and thickens.

Makes 3 (1-cup) servings

CURVES DIETERS: 8 carbs, 160 calories (per serving)
Free Foods in this recipe: celery, onion, bamboo shoots, bean sprouts, cabbage, snow peas, mushrooms, and garlic
Nutritional Information (per serving): Calories: 203, Fat: 13.5g, Saturated Fat: 2g, Protein: 3g, Carbohydrates: 18g, Fiber: 4g, Cholesterol: 0mg, Sodium: 516mg

LEMONY CAULIFLOWER

PREPARATION TIME: *20 minutes*

2 cups cauliflower florets

1 tablespoon butter

2 teaspoons lemon juice

1 tablespoon chopped fresh parsley

½ teaspoon lemon-pepper seasoning

1 tablespoon heavy cream

Steam cauliflower until tender. Melt butter in a medium skillet. Add lemon juice, parsley, and lemon-pepper seasoning. Bring to a boil. Stir in cream. Add cauliflower and stir, and cook 2 minutes, until sauce thickens.

Makes 2 (1-cup) servings

CURVES DIETERS: 0 carbs, 75 calories (per serving)

Free Foods in this recipe: cauliflower, lemon juice, and parsley

Nutritional Information (per serving): Calories: 101, Fat: 8.5g, Saturated Fat: 5.5g, Protein: 1g, Carbohydrates: 6g, Fiber: 3g, Cholesterol: 26mg, Sodium: 153mg

PARMESAN VEGETABLE STIR-FRY

PREPARATION TIME: *15 minutes*

½ onion, thinly sliced (approximately ¾ cup)

1 clove garlic, minced

1 tablespoon olive oil

½ cup sliced mushrooms

1 cup fresh spinach (packed)

1 tablespoon lemon juice

½ ounce (2 tablespoons) shredded Parmesan cheese

Saute onion and garlic in olive oil until soft. Add mushrooms and cook until soft. Add spinach. Toss well and saute very briefly. Sprinkle with lemon juice and Parmesan cheese. Serve hot.

Makes 1 serving

CURVES DIETERS: 0 carbs, 175 calories (per serving)

Free Foods in this recipe: onion, garlic, mushrooms, spinach, and lemon juice

Nutritional Information (per serving): Calories: 275, Fat: 17g, Saturated Fat: 0g, Protein: 8g, Carbohydrates: 22g, Fiber: 6g, Cholesterol: 10mg, Sodium: 1,189mg

SPICY ZUCCHINI BOATS

PREPARATION TIME: *35 minutes*

4 small zucchini

6 cups boiling, salted water

4 ounces light cream cheese, softened

½ cup (2 ounces) shredded pepper jack cheese

½ cup shredded Parmesan cheese

¼ teaspoon cayenne pepper

1 teaspoon dried chives

Medium-size bowl of ice

Preheat oven to 350 degrees. Slice zucchini in half lengthwise to make boats. Blanch zucchini in boiling, salted water for 2 minutes. Drain, then immediately immerse zucchini in an ice bath. Drain thoroughly, blotting excess water with paper towels. Using a knife or small spoon, carefully hollow out zucchini by removing some of its pulp. (Leave at least a ¼-inch wall.)

Combine cheeses, cayenne pepper, and chives in a mixing bowl. Stuff zucchini with cheese mixture. Place in a lightly greased baking dish. Bake for 8 to 10 minutes or until squash is heated through and cheese is melted.

Recipes

Makes 4 (2-piece) servings

CURVES DIETERS: 2 carbs, 195 calories (per serving)

Free Foods in this recipe: zucchini

Nutritional Information (per serving): Calories: 210, Fat: 16g, Saturated Fat: 7g, Protein: 13g, Carbohydrates: 5g, Fiber: 1g, Cholesterol: 48mg, Sodium: 476mg

FROZEN CHOCOLATE MOUSSE

PREPARATION TIME: *1 hour 30 minutes*

12 ounces silken tofu (soft)

½ cup semisweet chocolate chips

1½ ounces unsweetened chocolate

½ cup granular Splenda

¼ cup water

3 egg whites

¼ teaspoon salt

2 tablespoons heavy cream

1 teaspoon vanilla extract

Remove tofu from package and place between several layers of paper towels. Weight with a plate for at least 15 minutes to press excess water out of tofu. Place chocolate chips and unsweetened chocolate in a microwave-safe bowl. Cover and microwave 1 minute, or until melted. Stir well and set aside. Combine Splenda and water in a small saucepan and bring to a boil. Turn off heat under saucepan. In a medium bowl, beat egg whites and salt on high speed until stiff peaks form. Continue beating on high and pour hot Splenda syrup very slowly into beaten egg whites. Set meringue aside. Beat tofu, melted chocolate, heavy cream, and vanilla together until very smooth. Beat in half of meringue. Fold in remaining meringue. Line 8 cupcake pan wells with paper cupcake liners. Spoon approximately ¼ of mousse into each and pack down well. Cover with plastic wrap and freeze about 1 hour. Remove from cupcake pan (you may need to rub the bottom of the pan with a hot, wet washcloth to free the liners) and put into a freezer bag. Store in the freezer until ready to serve. Before serving, let frozen mousse sit at room temperature for 5 minutes before peeling off paper liner.

Makes 8 (¼-cup) servings

CURVES DIETERS: 9 carbs, 127 calories (per serving)
Free Foods in this recipe: none
Nutritional Information (per serving): Calories: 127, Fat: 7g, Saturated Fat: 1g, Protein: 7g, Carbohydrates: 9g, Fiber: 1g, Cholesterol: 5mg, Sodium: 161mg

ITALIAN SODA

PREPARATION TIME: *2 minutes*

4 ice cubes
¼ cup sugar-free fruit-flavored syrup
2 tablespoons heavy cream
Sugar-free lemon-lime-flavored sparkling water

Place ice cubes in a tall glass. Pour syrup over them. Pour in cream. Fill glass with sparkling water and stir well.

Makes 1 serving

CURVES DIETERS: 0 carbs, 100 calories (per serving)
Free Foods in this recipe: none
Nutritional Information (per serving): Calories: 100, Fat: 10g, Saturated Fat: 7g, Protein: 0g, Carbohydrates: 2g, Fiber: 0g, Cholesterol: 40mg, Sodium: 40mg

Recipes

STRAWBERRY-MANGO PROTEIN SHAKE

PREPARATION TIME: *5 minutes*

8 ounces 2% milk

1 tablespoon granular Splenda

½ scoop low-carb whey protein powder

¼ cup frozen strawberries (no sugar added)

¼ cup frozen mango chunks (no sugar added)

3 ice cubes

Pour milk into blender. Add Splenda and whey protein powder. Blend for 2 minutes. Add frozen fruit and ice cubes and blend 2 more minutes.

Makes 1 serving

CURVES DIETERS: 23 carbs, 206 calories (per serving)

Free Foods in this recipe: none

Nutritional Information (per serving): Calories: 206, Fat: 5g, Saturated Fat: 3g, Protein: 17g, Carbohydrates: 23g, Fiber: 0g, Cholesterol: 20mg, Sodium: 143mg

MULTIVITAMIN/MINERAL SUPPLEMENT SHOPPING LIST

Don't Leave Home Without This List

Take this list to the store with you when you purchase your multivitamin to make sure that you are getting everything that you need.

Basic Multivitamin/Mineral Formula

Vitamin A	10,000 RE	*not for pregnant women*
Vitamin C	1,000 mg	
Vitamin D	400 IU	*If you are taking a calcium supplement with vitamin D, as many women do, you will not need as much D in your multivitamin.*
Vitamin E	200–400 IU	
Vitamin B_1 (thiamine)	25 mg	
Vitamin B_2 (riboflavin)	25 mg	
Niacin	25 mg	
Vitamin B_6	40 mg	
Folic acid (folate)	400 mcg	
Vitamin B_{12}	200 mcg	
Calcium	1,000–1,500 mg	*Most women need to take a calcium supplement for bone support.*
Iron	4 mg	*Women with idiopathic hemochromatosis should not take a supplement with iron.*
Magnesium	100 mg	
Zinc	15 mg	
Selenium	70–200 mcg	
Copper	2 mg	
Manganese	5 mg	

| Chromium | 120–200 mcg |
| Potassium | 100 mg |

Additional Antioxidants and Phytochemicals

If these antioxidants are not already in your multivitamin, look for an antioxidant supplement that includes the following:

Alpha-lipoic acid	25 mg
Mixed citrus bioflavonoids	1,000 mg
Co-Q10	30 mg
Lutein	50 mg
N-acetyl cysteine (NAC)	100 mg
Lycopene	25 mg for women (100 mg for men)
Quercetin	50 mg

Essential Fatty Acids

If essential fatty acids are not already in your multivitamin/ mineral supplement, look for an essential fatty acid supplement containing omega-3, -6, and -9.

500–1,000 mg

Amino Acids

If amino acids are not already included in your multivitamin/ mineral supplement, look for an additional supplement that includes the following:

Multi-predigested amino acids   500–1,000 mg

DAILY MEAL PLANNER

PHASE 1

CARBOHYDRATE-SENSITIVE PLAN: DO NOT EXCEED 20 GRAMS
OF CARBOHYDRATES DAILY.

CALORIE-SENSITIVE PLAN: DO NOT EXCEED 1,200 CALORIES AND 60 GRAMS
OF CARBOHYDRATES DAILY.

	DAY _____	Carbs	Calories
Meal 1			
Meal 2			
Meal 3			
Meal 4			
Meal 5			
Meal 6			
	TOTALS		

	DAY _____	Carbs	Calories
Meal 1			
Meal 2			
Meal 3			
Meal 4			
Meal 5			
Meal 6			
	TOTALS		

	DAY _____	Carbs	Calories
Meal 1			
Meal 2			
Meal 3			
Meal 4			
Meal 5			
Meal 6			
	TOTALS		

	DAY _____	Carbs	Calories
Meal 1			
Meal 2			
Meal 3			
Meal 4			
Meal 5			
Meal 6			
	TOTALS		

	DAY _____	Carbs	Calories
Meal 1			
Meal 2			
Meal 3			
Meal 4			
Meal 5			
Meal 6			
	TOTALS		

PHASE 2

CARBOHYDRATE-SENSITIVE PLAN: DO NOT EXCEED 60 GRAMS
OF CARBOHYDRATES DAILY.

CALORIE-SENSITIVE PLAN: DO NOT EXCEED 1,600 CALORIES AND 60 GRAMS
OF CARBOHYDRATES DAILY.

	DAY _____	Carbs	Calories
Meal 1			
Meal 2			
Meal 3			
Meal 4			
Meal 5			
Meal 6			
	TOTALS		

	DAY _____	Carbs	Calories
Meal 1			
Meal 2			
Meal 3			
Meal 4			
Meal 5			
Meal 6			
	TOTALS		

	DAY _____	Carbs	Calories
Meal 1			
Meal 2			
Meal 3			
Meal 4			
Meal 5			
Meal 6			
	TOTALS		

	DAY _____	Carbs	Calories
Meal 1			
Meal 2			
Meal 3			
Meal 4			
Meal 5			
Meal 6			
	TOTALS		

	DAY _____	Carbs	Calories
Meal 1			
Meal 2			
Meal 3			
Meal 4			
Meal 5			
Meal 6			
	TOTALS		

PHASE 3:   RETRAINING YOUR METABOLISM CHART

STEP 1 · ESTABLISH YOUR LOW AND HIGH WEIGHT · Your current weight—that is, your post-diet weight before you go on Phase 3—is your *low* weight. Weigh yourself every morning before breakfast. Start eating normally. Within a day or two, you will notice a weight gain of about three to five pounds, depending on your body size. This is your *high* weight. Keep track of your weight daily on the following chart. Use a new chart each month. Your goal is to stay between your low weight and your high weight, and not gain any more weight.

Please note that some of you may have monthly weight fluctuations due to your menstrual periods. Women who are prone to bloating may gain an additional three pounds a few days before the start of their menstrual cycles. If you know that you are prone to gain a few pounds every month before your period, simply subtract the extra monthly weight gain from your true high weight so you don't go back to Phase 1 needlessly. In other words, those extra "period pounds" don't count.

STEP 2 · DON'T EXCEED YOUR HIGH WEIGHT · As soon as you hit your high weight, go back to Phase 1 to burn off the fat. On Phase 1, you will quickly lose the water and the fat, probably within a day or two. When you are back to your low weight, resume normal eating. *Try not to stay on Phase 1 for more than 72 hours, or you will stimulate the production of starvation hormones, which will further depress your metabolism.*

STEP 3 · KEEP GOING · Weigh yourself daily. Whenever you reach your high weight, go back to Phase 1 to burn off the fat. Try not to stay on Phase 1 for more than 72 hours—as soon as you reach your low weight, resume normal eating. Over a 30-day period, you will notice that you are dieting about 6 to 8 days of the month and eating normally the other 20. As your metabolism rises, it will take longer and longer to gain those extra pounds back. Within two or three months, most women are able to eat normally for weeks at a time and must go back to Phase 1 for only one or two days a month to maintain their weight. If your metabolism is a bit slower, it may take longer. If you party a lot and continually exceed 2,500 to 3,000 calories daily, you will find that you have to go back on Phase 1 more often to burn off the extra pounds. When you resume eating normally, you will soon be back on schedule.

SAMPLE CHART

Weight	1	2	3	4	5	6	7	8	9	10	11	12	13	14	15	16	17	18	19	20	21	22	23	24	25	26	27	28	29
HIGH																													
140		X							X									X											
139		X					X	X							X	X	X											X	X
138			X	X		X				X		X	X	X					X	X			X	X	X	X	X		
LOW 137	X				X						X										X	X							

Days

Your low weight is 137. Your high weight is 140. Keep track of your weight every day on the Phase 3 chart. Use a new chart for each month. You can eat normally until you reach your high weight (140), which, in this sample Phase 3 chart, occurs on Day 3. When you reach your high weight, go back on Phase 1 until you get down to your low weight (137), which happens here on Day 5. From Day 5, you can eat normally until you reach your high weight (140), which happens here on Day 9. When you reach your high weight, go back on Phase 1 until you reach your low weight (137), which happens here on Day 11.

From Day 11, you can eat normally until Day 18, when you hit your high weight (140) and must go back on Phase 1. Stay on Phase 1 until you reach your low weight (137) on Day 21. From Days 21 to 31, you are eating normally. If you were following this sample chart, you would be eating normally until the next time you hit your high weight of 140. Notice that each time you cycle in and out of Phase 1, you are able to eat normally for a longer period of time before you have to go back on Phase 1. Why? Your metabolism is increasing as your body rids itself of its starvation hormones.

You can photocopy additional charts directly from this book, or you can download them from my website, www.curvesinternational.com.

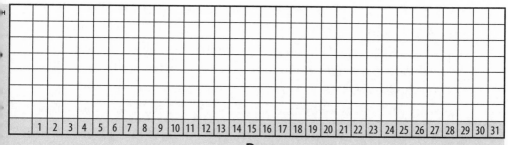

Days

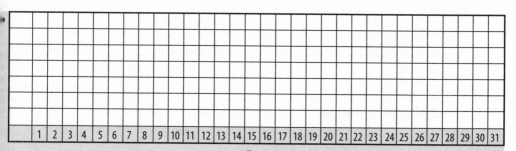

Days

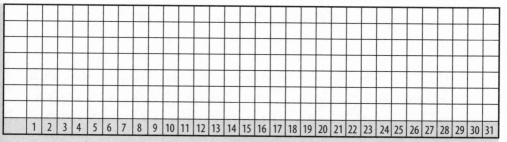

Days

THE METABOLIC TUNE-UP TRACKING CHART

STEP 1 · ESTABLISH YOUR LOW AND HIGH WEIGHTS · Your current weight—that is, your post-diet weight before you go on Phase 3—is your *low* weight. Record it on the following chart. Weigh yourself every morning before breakfast. Start eating normally. Within a day or two, you will notice a weight gain of about three to five pounds, depending on your body size. This is your *high* weight. Keep track of your weight daily on your Metabolic Tune-Up Tracking Chart. Use a new chart each month. Your goal is to stay between your low weight and your high weight, and not gain any more weight.

Please note that some of you may have monthly weight fluctuations due to your menstrual periods. Women who are prone to bloating may gain an additional three pounds a few days before the start of their menstrual cycles. If you know that you are prone to gain a few pounds every month before your period, simply subtract the extra monthly weight gain from your true high weight so you don't go back to Phase 1 needlessly. In other words, those extra "period pounds" don't count.

STEP 2 · DON'T EXCEED YOUR HIGH WEIGHT · As soon as you hit your high weight, go to Phase 1 to burn off the fat. *Try not to stay on Phase 1 for more than 72 hours, or you will stimulate the production of starvation hormones, which will further depress your metabolism.* When you are back to your low weight, resume normal eating.

STEP 3 · KEEP GOING · Weigh yourself daily. Whenever you reach your high weight, go back to Phase 1 to burn off the fat. Try not to stay on Phase 1 for more than 72 hours—as soon as you reach your low weight, resume normal eating. Don't assume that if you are taking weight off easily, it means that it's time to go back on a weight-loss diet. If you start dieting now, you will quickly plateau and end up right back where you started.

As your metabolic rate increases, it will take longer and longer to gain those extra pounds back. You are ready to resume your weight-loss diet when you can eat normally for four weeks or so at a time without gaining weight and only need to go to Phase 1 for one or two days a month.

What next? When you have completed your Metabolic Tune-Up, if you have more than 20 pounds to lose, go back to Phase 1 for two weeks and then move on to Phase 2. If you have less than 20 pounds to lose, go to Phase 1 for one week and then move on to Phase 2.

SAMPLE CHART

GH																															
150			X							X								X												X
149		X				X	X	X								X	X						X	X	X	X	
148	X				X					X	X	X							X	X	X						
147			X					X	X								X		X								
146	X			X					X						X												
	1	2	3	4	5	6	7	8	9	10	11	12	13	14	15	16	17	18	19	20	21	22	23	24	25	26	27	28	29	30	31

D a y s

Your current weight (your low weight) is 146. Your high weight is 150. Keep track of your weight every day on the Phase 3 chart. Use a new chart for each month. You can eat normally until you reach your high weight (150), which, in this sample Phase 3 chart, occurs on Day 4. When you reach your high weight, go back on Phase 1 until you get down to your low weight (146), which happens here on Day 6. From Day 6, you can eat normally until you reach your high weight (150), which happens here on Day 11. When you reach your high weight, go back on Phase 1 until you reach your low weight (146), which happens here on Day 14.

From Day 14, you can eat normally until Day 20, when you hit your high weight (150) and must go back on Phase 1. Stay on Phase 1 until you reach your low weight (146), which happens here on Day 22. From Day 22, you are eating normally. If you were following this sample chart, you would eat normally until the next time you hit your high weight of 150 at Day 31. Notice that each time you cycle in and out of Phase 1 you are able to eat normally for a longer period of time before you have to go back on Phase 1. Why? Your metabolism is increasing as your body rids itself of its starvation hormones.

When you are able to go for 3 to 4 weeks at a time without gaining weight, you are ready to resume your weight-loss program.

You can photocopy additional charts directly from this book, or you can download them from my website, www.curvesinternational.com.

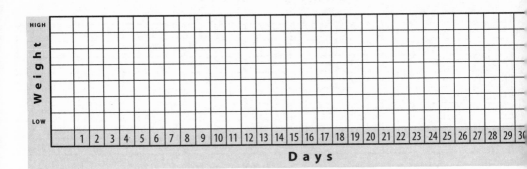

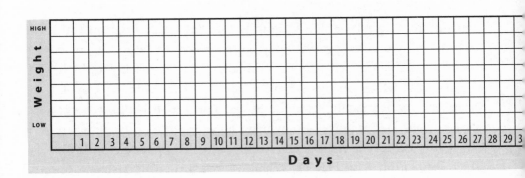

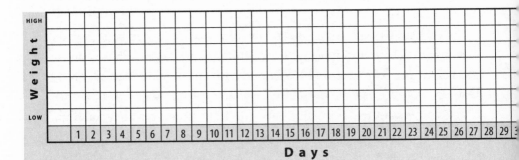

WEEKLY PROGRESS REPORT

Write your beginning weight in the top box in the left column, and enter one-pound decreases down the column. Place an X in the corresponding weekly weight amounts. Place your goal weight in the goal box. This graph will help you visualize your success.

SAMPLE CHART

Start								Goal
	Week 1	Week 2	Week 3	Week 4	Week 5	Week 6	Week 7	
eight								
85	X							
84								
83								
82		X						
81								
80			X					

Start								Goal
	Week 1	Week 2	Week 3	Week 4	Week 5	Week 6	Week 7	
eight								

BIBLIOGRAPHY

Adlercreutz, H., et al. "Western Diet and Western Disease: Some Hormonal and Biochemical Mechanisms and Associations." *Scandinavian Journal of Clinical and Laboratory Investigation* 50, Supplement 201 (1990).

———. "Dietary Phyto-estrogens and Menopause in Japan." *The Lancet* 342 (May 16, 1992).

"Alternatives to Hormone Replacement Therapy." The North American Menopause Society, Mayfield, Ohio (July 11, 2002), www.menopause.org.

Anderson, J. W. "Dietary Fiber and Diabetes: A Comprehensive Review and Practical Application." *Journal of the American Diabetic Association* 87 (September 1987).

———. "Dietary Fiber: Diabetes and Obesity." *American Journal of Gastroenterology* 81 (October 10, 1986).

Anderson, R. A., et al. "Elevated Intakes of Supplemental Chromium Improve Glucose and Insulin Variables in Individuals with Type II Diabetes." *Diabetes* 46 (1997).

Ascherio, A., et al. "Health Effects of Transfatty Acids." *American Journal of Clinical Nutrition* 66, Supplement (1997).

Bendich, A., and L. Langseth. "The Health Effects of Vitamin C Supplementation: A Review." *Journal of the American College of Nutrition* 14:124–36.

Brown, P., ed. *Understanding and Applying Medical Anthropology.* Mountain View, Calif.: Mayfield Publishing Company, 1998.

Cockburn, A. *Mummies, Disease and Ancient Cultures.* Cambridge: Cambridge University Press, 1980.

Copper, K. *Advanced Nutritional Therapies.* Nashville, Tenn.: Thomas Nelson Publishers, 1998.

Eaton, S. B., et al. "Paleolithic Nutrition Revisited: A Twelve-Year Retrospective on Its Nature and Implications." *European Journal of Clinical Nutrition* 51 (1997).

Fuchs, Jürgen, et al. *Lipoic Acid in Health and Disease.* Marcel Dekker, New York: 1997.

Fumento, M. *The Fat of the Land.* New York: Viking, 1997.

Grady, D., et al., for the HERS Research Group. "Cardiovascular Disease Outcomes During 6.8 Years of Hormone Therapy: Heart and Estrogen/Progestin Replacement Study Follow-up (HERS II)." *Journal of the American Medical Association* 288 (2002).

Guidelines for Exercise During Pregnancy. American College of Obstetricians and Gynecologists. Based on an interview with Dr. Wayne Westcott.

Hulley, S., et al., for the HERS Research Group. "Non-Cardiovascular Disease Outcomes During 6.8 Years of Hormone Therapy: Heart and Estrogen/ Progestin Replacement Study Follow-up (HERS II)." *Journal of the American Medical Association* 288 (2002).

Kelly, G. "Clinical Applications of N-acetylcysteine." *Alternative Medicine Review* Vol. 3:2 (April 1998): 114–27.

Legato, M. L., and C. Colman, *The Female Heart: The Truth About Women and Coronary Artery Disease.* New York: Simon & Schuster, 1991.

Losoncszy, K. G., et al., "Vitamin E and Vitamin C Supplement Use and Risk of All Cause and Coronary Heart Disease and Mortality in Older Persons: The Established Populations for Epidemiologic Studies of the Elderly." *American Journal of Clinical Nutrition* 64 (1996).

Ludwig, D. S., et al. "Dietary Fiber, Weight Gain, and Cardiovascular Disease Risk Factors in Young Adults." *Journal of the American Medical Association* 283 (October 27, 1999).

Manson, J. E., et al. "Body Weight and Mortality Among Women." *The New England Journal of Medicine* 33:11 (September 14, 1995).

Miller, W. C., et al. "Dietary Fat, Sugar and Fiber Predict Body Fat Content." *Journal of the American Dietetic Association* 94 (June 6, 1994).

Mokdad, A. H., et al. "The Spread of the Obesity Epidemic in the United States, 1991–1998." *Journal of the American Medical Association* 282 (October 27, 1999).

Mowrey, D. *The Scientific Validation of Herbal Medicine.* New Canaan, Conn.: Keats Publishing, 1986.

National Task Force on the Prevention and Treatment of Obesity. "Weight Cycling." *Journal of the American Medical Association* 272:15 (October 19, 1994).

Packer, L., and C. Colman, *The Antioxidant Miracle: Your Complete Plan for Total Health and Healing.* New York: John Wiley & Sons, 1999.

"Questions and Answers About Black Cohosh and the Symptoms of Menopause." National Institutes of Health, Office of Dietary Supplements, National Center for Complementary and Alternative Medicine. http://ods.od.nih.gov/factsheets/blackcohosh.html.

"Rating the Diets." *Consumer Reports* 58 (June 6, 1993).

Roberts, S. *Personal Training Manual.* American Council on Exercise (1996).

Rooney, B. L., et al. "Excess Pregnancy Weight Gain and Long-Term Obesity: One Decade Later." *Obstetrics and Gynecology* 100 (August, 2002): 245–52.

Seidel, J. C. "Obesity in Europe: Scaling an Epidemic." *International Journal of Obesity,* 19 Supplement 3 (September 1995).

Simopoulos, A. "Omega-3 Fatty Acids in Health and Disease and in Growth and Development." *American Journal of Clinical Nutrition* 54 (1991): 438–63.

Somer, E. *The Nutrition Desk Reference.* New York: Keats Publishing, 1995.

Strause, L., et al. "Spinal Bone Loss in Postmenopausal Women Supplemented with Calcium and Trace Minerals." *Journal of Nutrition* 124 (1994).

Theodosaskis, J. *The Arthritis Cure.* New York: St. Martin's Press, 1997.

"The Rockefeller Study." *New England Journal of Medicine* (March 9, 1995).

U.S. Bureau of Census. *Statistical Abstract* 147, table 225 (Washington, D.C., 1995).

U.S. Department of Agriculture, Agriculture Research Service. "What We Eat in America: 1994–96." Results from the 1994–96 Continuing Survey of Food Intakes by Individuals (1996).

VERIS Newsletter (La Grange, Ill.: VERIS Research Information Service).

Wadden, T. A., et al. "Effects of Weight Cycling on the Resting Energy Expenditure and Body Composition of Obese Women." *International Journal of Eating Disorders* 19 (January 1996).

Whiting, K. S. *How to Naturally Control Diabetes and Hypoglycemia.* San Diego, Calif.: Institute of Nutritional Science, 1998.

————. *Well at Any Age.* San Diego, Calif.: Institute of Nutritional Science, 2000.

INDEX

ABOUT THE AUTHORS

Twenty-seven years ago, at the age of twenty, Gary Heavin began his career as a nutrition counselor and fitness instructor. Over the years, he has personally coached thousands of women through the process of attaining optimal weight and health. He and his wife, Diane, perfected the Curves concepts at their first location in Harlingen, Texas, in 1992. The regimen was simple: a complete thirty-minute workout three days a week and a temporary dieting method that produced permanent results in a supportive environment. The concept was an overwhelming success, and in 1995, the first Curves franchise opened. In just eight years, Curves has grown from just one franchise to almost 6,000. Curves is now the world's largest fitness franchise, and the fastest-growing franchise organization of any kind.

Curves™

GUEST PASS

FREE

1 WEEK MEMBERSHIP *

Call

1-888-300-0274

or go to our website at

www.curvesinternational.com

to locate the facility nearest you.

*May be exchanged for a special first visit discount, one per person, new members only, must be 18 years or older. Valid at participating locations. Void where prohibited.

The **power** TO **AMAZE** YOURSELF.